Secrets of Dragon Gate

*Ancient Taoist Practices for Health, Wealth,
and the Art of Sexual Yoga*

Dr. Steven Liu *and* Jonathan Blank

JEREMY P. TARCHER/PENGUIN
a member of Penguin Group (USA) Inc.
New York

JEREMY P. TARCHER/PENGUIN
Published by the Penguin Group
Penguin Group (USA) Inc., 375 Hudson Street, New York, New York 10014, USA • Penguin Group
(Canada), 90 Eglinton Avenue East, Suite 700, Toronto, Ontario M4P 2Y3, Canada (a division of
Pearson Penguin Canada Inc.) • Penguin Books Ltd, 80 Strand, London WC2R 0RL, England •
Penguin Ireland, 25 St Stephen's Green, Dublin 2, Ireland (a division of Penguin Books Ltd) •
Penguin Group (Australia), 250 Camberwell Road, Camberwell, Victoria 3124, Australia (a division of
Pearson Australia Group Pty Ltd) • Penguin Books India Pvt Ltd, 11 Community Centre, Panchsheel Park,
New Delhi–110 017, India • Penguin Group (NZ), 67 Apollo Drive, Rosedale, North Shore 0632,
New Zealand (a division of Pearson New Zealand Ltd) • Penguin Books (South Africa) (Pty) Ltd,
24 Sturdee Avenue, Rosebank, Johannesburg 2196, South Africa

Penguin Books Ltd, Registered Offices: 80 Strand, London WC2R 0RL, England

All calligraphy in this book was created by Dr. Steven Liu. The Five Celestial Guardian illustrations
are by Sharon Liu (Dr. Liu's daughter). The exercise images were created by Stephanie Murray from
photographs taken by Colby Devitt. The Five Element chart was created by Fiely Matias.

Most Tarcher/Penguin books are available at special quantity discounts for bulk purchase for
sales promotions, premiums, fund-raising, and educational needs. Special books or book excerpts
also can be created to fit specific needs. For details, write Penguin Group (USA) Inc.
Special Markets, 375 Hudson Street, New York, NY 10014.

Library of Congress Cataloging-in-Publication Data

Liu, Steven, date.
Secrets of Dragon Gate: ancient Taoist practices for health, wealth, and the art of sexual yoga /
Steven Liu and Jonathan Blank.
p.   cm.
ISBN 978-1-58542-843-4
1. Quan zhen jiao.   2. Taoism.   I. Blank, Jonathan.   II. Title.
BL1943.C55L58   2011   2010039336
299.5'149—dc22

Printed in the United States of America
1   3   5   7   9   10   8   6   4   2

Book design by Meighan Cavanaugh

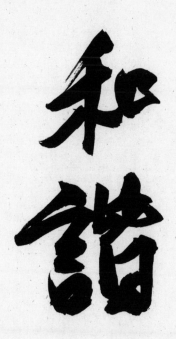

Harmony

CONTENTS

PREFACE

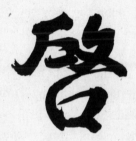

Begin

The source of all things is in the Tao.
It is a treasure for the good, and a refuge for all in need.
On auspicious occasions, when gifts are sent, rather than sending
  horses or jade, send the teachings of the Tao.

—LAO TZU

I first became interested in Taoism many years ago when, as a boy,
I read amazing tales of legendary Taoist immortals who mastered the five elements and achieved superhuman abilities. These

"immortals" started their lives as ordinary people, but with diligent practice they transformed themselves into magical beings who existed on a higher plane of consciousness. According to Taoist philosophy, the immortals' path is available to anyone who wishes to pursue it.

Spurred on by the stories, I dreamed of becoming a Taoist immortal too, and so I set out on a course of study that has continued throughout my life. Along the way, one of the key things I've learned is that Taoism provides excellent long-term solutions for maintaining optimum health and vitality as well as a powerful way to understand and make the most of reality.

Over the years, I trained with many remarkable Taoist masters both in the United States and Asia. Then, in the mid-1990s, I met Dr. Liu at his Taoist temple in, fittingly enough, Temple City, California. I was immediately struck by his kind, laid-back, and engaging manner and the way he easily breaks into laughter. He has been studying Taoism since he was a boy and is now the fourteenth-generation master of the Taiwanese branch of the Dragon Gate school of Taoism, a complete system for applying traditional Taoist methods to enhance every aspect of a person's life. It's an approach that enables people to pursue a path that is simultaneously metaphysical and pragmatic, something that strongly appealed to me.

The Dragon Gate school of Taoism is a nearly eight-hundred-year-old system of Chinese philosophy, martial arts, meditation, magic, and mysticism. It is a very mysterious tradition, little known in the West, that provides a practical system for creating a magical Taoist reality—even if you live in a bustling modern-day metropolis. It does this by combining all the best elements of Taoism including:

- meditation practices to develop your mental capabilities
- chi-gung (energy work) and martial arts exercises for health and longevity
- sexual yoga and dream yoga that reach deep into Taoism's shamanic roots
- philosophy, based on the Yi Jing (I Ching), or Book of Changes, and the five elements, that provides profound insight into the nature of reality
- divination methods for developing your intuition

Best of all, the methods are quite simple, so anyone can practice them and reap the benefits, regardless of health or age.

I have been studying with Dr. Liu for many years now and have seen him teach and help hundreds of people. He has mastered all aspects of the Dragon Gate system. Put simply, he is the real deal. The information in this book has been handed down directly through the centuries to Dr. Liu, who has in turn passed them on to me. I have also incorporated other sources of Taoist information that I have learned over the years where I felt it would enhance the text.

In *Secrets of Dragon Gate*, I have attempted to distill Dragon Gate Taoism into its most usable form, so the average person can take full advantage of this ancient and secretive tradition to attain optimum health, bring abundance into their lives, and find lasting happiness. I chose to write it because I wish I had been able to find a similar book when I started on my path.

I wish you bold flowing as you pursue your own path.

Jonathan Blank

A note on Chinese transliteration used in this book: I have used both traditional Wade-Giles transliteration as well as the more modern pinyin. I did this because I felt that certain words are more commonly recognized in Wade-Giles, such as Tao (Dao) *and* chi (qi). *I apologize if this inconsistency is disturbing to any readers.*

SECRETS OF DRAGON GATE
EXERCISES

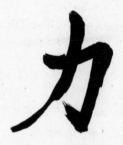

Power

Exercise Index

- The Microcosmic Orbit Exercise
- The Golden Stove Exercise

Guidelines for Practicing the Exercises in This Book

Be still like a great mountain.
Move like a flowing river.

—CHANG SAN-FENG, CREATOR OF TAI CHI

Since Dragon Gate is a Taoist system, the simple answer to how you should practice is to do that which feels natural. Of course, everyone has a different idea of what is "natural," and many people appreciate guidance, especially at the beginning, to get started on their way. It is in that spirit that the following suggestions are made. But please be aware that all the suggestions in this chapter are just that—suggestions. If something does not feel right to you, then you need to adapt the instructions for your own comfort. It is also important to remember that the exercises presented in this book are easy to do. They should never cause pain or discomfort. If you do feel any pain or discomfort, stop doing the exercise.

- **Clothing:** Wear loose, comfortable clothes that do not bind the body or constrict breathing. Remember that your energy channels are like a garden hose. When you squeeze the hose, you constrict the flow. Wear clothing that keeps you warm enough to practice but not so warm that you sweat excessively. As for footwear, soft, flat, rubber-soled shoes that provide good traction are best. You can also practice barefoot if you have strong feet and ankles and weather permits. Barefoot practice can be especially good when you are practicing on a natural surface with a direct connection to the earth, such as grass.

- **Location:** Find a place where you can be comfortable. This can be inside or outside, but you should make sure there are no major distractions such as noise, weather, etc., that could interfere with your practice. It's a good idea to turn off the phone and anything else that may make noise and disturb you. Make sure the floor or ground you practice on is flat. The ideal location is outside (when the weather is good) in peaceful, natural surroundings. However, any location that is quiet and comfortable is good. Avoid rooms that are air conditioned or that have a fan blowing toward you.

- **Timing:** You can practice at any time of day. Typically early morning, when you are fresh and reinvigorated, is an excellent time. But really any time of day is good. A lot depends on your natural rhythms and your schedule. Find what works for you. Make sure to wait at least one hour after eating a meal before practicing. Drink a cup of warm water before practicing because it helps your chi (internal energy) start to circulate. Conversely, don't drink anything cold an hour before and an hour after practice.

- **Duration:** Try to do at least 10 to 15 minutes of practice 4 to 5 days a week. However, you can do these exercises for much longer and as many times a week as you like. Unlike weight lifting or other strenuous exercises that require a rest period, the exercises in this book can be (and ideally are) practiced daily. Regular, short periods of practice are far superior to infrequent, long periods of practice. The important thing is consistency. So find an amount of practice that works for you and do it regularly.

- **Body position:** The key point to remember for most exercises is to keep your back straight and to find a position that feels comfortable and relaxed.

  - When sitting: ensure that the chair you are sitting on allows you to be at a seated height where your knees can be comfortably bent at a 90- to 100-degree angle. If the chair is too short, you can use pillows to elevate your buttocks. Keep your head straight and look straight ahead. Your chin should be parallel with the ground. Keep your back straight, but not tense. Allow your shoulders and elbows to hang completely relaxed. Place your hands on your thighs (palms up or down). Your feet should be parallel or pointed slightly outward, shoulder-width apart. You may keep your eyes half open or closed, depending on which is most comfortable for you.

  - When standing: keep your back straight, but not tense. Your feet should be parallel or pointed slightly outward, shoulder-width apart. The knees should be directly over the feet. Allow your shoulders and elbows to hang completely relaxed. The feeling of standing meditation is similar to how you feel when sitting on the edge of a bar stool. You may keep your eyes half open or closed, depending on which is most comfortable for you.

- **Breathing:** Breathe slowly and deeply through the nose (unless you are unable to breathe through your nose due to illness or other factors, in which case you should breathe through your mouth). Keep your mouth closed with the tip of the tongue against the roof of the mouth just behind the top teeth. When you breathe in your abdomen should expand, and when you breathe out your abdomen should contract. Once you have established the pattern of breathing from your abdomen, try not to focus on it and just breathe naturally. It is important to remember never to hold your breath.

- **Motion:** For any exercise that involves motion (unless otherwise specified in the specific instructions for that exercise), move very slowly, smoothly, and evenly. Do not rush the exercises. Maintain a consistent pace throughout. Try to feel the air as a medium that you are moving through—like water—not just empty space. Avoid sudden stops and starts. Keep your movements soft and rounded and avoid hard edges. Stay relaxed and exert no muscular force.

TIPS ON RELAXATION

It's very easy to tell yourself to relax, but much harder to actually relax on command. In fact, the act of instructing yourself to relax is often stress-inducing. So the best way to relax is to shift your focus to something else . . . something that makes you relax. This can vary a lot depending on the person, but below are several ideas of ways to relax.

Suggestions for Relaxing the Body

- Take three very deep breaths, filling your lungs completely on inhale and expelling all the air on exhale. Do this calmly and slowly (don't hyperventilate).

- Keep a soft smile on your face. The expression of a soft smile immediately makes you more relaxed.
- Try to capture the feeling you get when you completely relax your body right before you urinate. You have to relax an extra amount to allow yourself to urinate, and you can use that same feeling to help you relax.
- Imagine yourself floating down a river.
- Imagine yourself taking a hot shower.
- Focus on any area of the body where you feel tension. Mentally send heat energy to that area until you feel it relax.

Suggestions for Relaxing the Mind

- Count your breaths. This is perhaps the most basic method for relaxation. Simply count your breaths. It's that simple. And it works.
- Think of a beautiful, serene place you've been such as the beach, a park, a mountain, or a forest. This can be any place that you associate with relaxation.
- Think of something that makes you feel happy and secure. This is similar to visualizing a beautiful place, but offers another approach.
- Think of something (a person, event, or time in your life) that brings true joy to you.
- Focus on your breathing. You can also count your breaths.
- Count backward from one hundred, slowly and steadily. If all else fails, this will work.
- Listen to the sounds you can hear, from those nearest or loudest, to those farthest away or faintest.

- Observe your thoughts. Make no effort to stifle your thoughts. Just watch them flow by as though they are floating on a river and you are standing peacefully on the riverbank watching them go by.
- Mentally light a fire in your mind and allow it to burn up any thoughts that pass through.
- Say the meditation number (from Chapter 9, "Advanced Alchemy") to yourself.

First Gate: What Is Dragon Gate Taoism?

A BRIEF HISTORY OF THE EXTRAORDINARY DRAGON GATE SCHOOL OF TAOISM

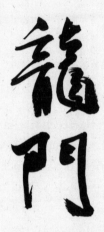

Dragon Gate

There was a gorge, known as the Dragon Gate, and legend had it that if a carp succeeded in jumping through the Dragon Gate it would emerge as a dragon.

—FROM *Seven Taoist Masters*

Please take the time now to enjoy a brief moment of meditative contemplation before you proceed with this chapter. It will help you to maximize your enjoyment of the chapter and retain more of the information. Simply make yourself comfortable, close your eyes, and take 3 very deep breaths. Now you are ready to begin.

Are You Ready to Become an Alchemist?

When I let go of who I am, I become who I might be.

—LAO TZU

Perhaps you've heard of the legendary attempts by medieval alchemists to turn base metals, such as lead, into gold. There are generally two interpretations of this alchemy. Some view these experiments as the first steps in the science of chemistry. Others see the alchemy as a metaphor for spiritual development and transmutation that is as relevant today as it was thousands of years ago. In this transformational process the practitioner turns his or her normal physical body (lead) into a magical body of energy (gold). This second interpretation is the one that applies to the Taoist alchemy that lies at the heart of Dragon Gate Taoism and is the subject of this book.

The Taoist focus on energy development, longevity, and enlightenment led to the invention of its own fascinating and highly secretive system of internal alchemy that also used the metaphor of turning lead into gold. In Taoist alchemy the practitioner converts their physical essence into spirit and ultimately the Tao itself. In this process, you learn to free the flow of chi, or internal energy, within your own body and synchronize it with the flow of energy in the universe. This opens new channels of energy and information while simultaneously slowing or even reversing the aging process.

This book provides you with a wide variety of techniques and exercises that you can use to follow the Taoist path and pursue the alchemy in your everyday life. In the Taoist tradition, *Secrets of Dragon Gate* provides you with ways to apply the alchemy to all aspects of your life—waking, sleeping, eating, exercising, lovemaking, and so on. The exercises and traditions in this book have been handed down from generation to generation and then honed and improved over the years with the input of many great masters.

Of course, anyone writing a book on Taoism faces the same conundrum described by Lao Tzu, the author of the quintessential Taoist philosophical manual the *Tao Te Ching*, who wrote, "The Tao that can be spoken of is not the eternal Tao" and "He who knows does not speak, and he who speaks does not know." So how does one write a book about a system of physical, spiritual, and psychological development when the very founder stated that those who know don't speak?

Naturally, Lao Tzu, as the author of a book on Taoism, must have faced this same question. It seems likely that Lao Tzu's cautionary words are directed more toward the readers than the writers of Taoist books and are meant to serve as a reminder for all those who wish to pursue the Tao that knowledge of the Tao must ultimately come from personal experience.

A Brief Overview of Taoism

Taoism, in its broadest sense, is the search for truth and reality. In
a narrower sense, it is the original knowledge tradition of China.
—LIU I-MING, TAOIST SCHOLAR, EIGHTEENTH CENTURY,
Awakening to the Tao

Taoism (pronounced dow-ism) refers to a variety of philosophical
and religious traditions and concepts that developed in China more
than twenty-five hundred years ago. Its roots can be traced to prehistoric shamanic folk religions. Lao Tzu is traditionally regarded
as the founder of Taoism, though there is no proof that a person
named Lao Tzu actually existed. He received imperial recognition
as a divinity in the second century A.D., and Taoism gained official
status in China during the Tang dynasty (A.D. 618–907).

The word *Tao* roughly translates as "path" or "way" and it can be
thought of as the flow of the universe, or the force behind the
natural order. At its core is the belief that humans are a microcosm
of the universe and that we are therefore able to gain knowledge of
the universe by understanding ourselves.

It is very difficult to characterize Taoism because it was not a
tradition whose leaders articulated an orthodox belief system. Nor
did they try to impose a rigid set of ideas about what Taoism is.
Taoism has never been a unified religion, but has rather consisted
of numerous teachings from many different sources and has often
been combined with Buddhism and Confucianism—the other two
primary philosophical/religious systems in China.

This eclecticism stems in part from the fact that Taoists did not
generally regard themselves as followers of a single religious community with a single set of teachings or practices. Unlike Christianity,

Confucianism, or Buddhism, Taoism did not grow out of supposedly divinely inspired teachings of a single leader. And since there were no original teachings or community, Taoists throughout history never felt obliged to make their beliefs and practices adhere to any particular standard.

Consequently there are many different schools of Taoism, and it is impossible to identify specific ideas or practices that are generally agreed upon by all Taoists. With the understanding that any description of Taoism is a generalization and that there will always be exceptions, there are still a number of core beliefs that the majority of schools share. We can divide Taoist practice into four general categories:

Philosophy: The first is Taoist philosophy, rooted in the teachings of Lao Tzu and Chuang Tzu, the two great philosophical masters of the tradition. This philosophy focuses on living in harmony with nature, human/universe correspondences, vitality, peace, emptiness, wu wei (effortless action), liberty, and spontaneity. This category also includes the core Taoist concepts of yin/yang, the ideas expressed in the Book of Changes and the Chinese five elements (wood, fire, earth, metal, water).

Health: The second is the Taoist pursuit of health and longevity. This part of Taoism includes the alchemical tradition mentioned above and also focuses on the development of chi (qi, or internal energy), health, Taoist martial arts (such as tai chi), Chinese medicine, and immortality.

Ethics: The third is ethics, a tradition strongly influenced by Confucianism, which emphasizes the importance of good deeds, and

Buddhism, which emphasizes the primary universal law of karma. This aspect of Taoism focuses on the Three Jewels of the Tao: compassion, moderation, and humility.

Esoteric Practices: The fourth is a general category that encompasses a variety of esoteric practices including ancestor worship, astrology, and other forms of divination, gardening, art (including calligraphy), vegetarian cuisine, feng shui, dream yoga, and sexual yoga.

Naturally, elements of the different categories overlap, and in typical Taoist fashion, they are meant to work as a whole and not as individual pieces—something you will see embodied in this book.

Over the years the influence of Taoism on Chinese culture has waxed and waned depending on who was in power at the time. But in recent times, Taoist practitioners traveled to the West and brought their knowledge and beliefs to a culture that has welcomed it. In the past several decades, hundreds of Taoist texts have been translated into English for the first time. In many ways there has never been a better time to study this ancient and fascinating tradition.

Enter Dragon Gate Taoism

The Tao is near and people seek it far away.

—MENCIUS

Dragon Gate Taoism is a nearly eight-hundred-year-old Chinese school of philosophy, exercise, arts, and sciences designed to guide its practitioners to a long life marked by excellent health combined with both spiritual and material abundance. Many of its esoteric practices have been closely guarded secrets for centuries.

Dragon Gate is an offshoot of the Complete Reality (Quan-Zhen or Ch'üan-chen) school of Taoism, which became popular by integrating elements of Buddhism and Confucianism. Complete Reality Taoism eventually spread throughout China during the Middle Ages and still continues to be popular today.

Complete Reality Taoism is generally divided into Southern and Northern branches. The Dragon Gate school is part of the Northern branch. The history of Dragon Gate is filled with apocryphal tales of great masters, often called "immortals" who led lives of self-discovery, magic, and mystery. (Those who achieve the highest levels of Taoist enlightenment are often referred to as "immortals" and it is believed that they can give up and retake human form at will.) While the true evolution of Dragon Gate Taoism cannot be known, the commonly accepted story goes something like this . . .

Lao Tzu (Laozi) who, according to the legend, lived in the sixth century B.C., passed his teachings on before he mysteriously departed from society. Over the years the tradition was passed from master to student in an uninterrupted succession until finally passing to Wang Xuanpu (Han dynasty, 206 B.C.–220 A.D.), a Taoist adept who practiced the golden elixir internal alchemy for spiritual development.

Wang then passed the teachings down to Chung-li Ch'uan, a famous general who lost his way in the mountains one day and met the reclusive Wang. The general was so impressed with the Taoist master that he gave up his military life to become a wandering seeker. These two men are considered the first two patriarchs of the Complete Reality school and, as is typical of the Taoist tradition, they reappear in different times in history to pass their teachings on to a new generation—since in the Taoist view of reality a great master is able to give up and retake human form at will.

This is how, according to the story, several hundred years later, during the Tang dynasty (A.D. 618–907), Chung-li met Lu Dongbin. At the time Lu was a young man planning for a life in the Chinese civil service. Instead, Chung-li led Lu to follow a path that resulted in him becoming perhaps the most famous of all Taoist "immortals." Lu Dongbin is revered today as a great scholar, poet, swordsman, and master of Taoist alchemy who emphasized the importance of inner cultivation and the attainment of spiritual immortality.

The next patriarch leading up to the development of the Dragon Gate school was Wang Chongyang who was born to a wealthy family in Shaanxi province at the end of the Northern Song dynasty (960–1127). He was a respected scholar and military officer, but was always dogged by a feeling of deep dissatisfaction with his life. Eventually he abandoned his family and career and became a wandering seeker whose unusual behavior led him to be nicknamed "Mad Wang." "Who can become an immortal without a touch of madness!" he is supposed to have said.

One day, while practicing in the mountains he fell in with two other wanderers who turned out to be Chung-li Ch'uan and Lu Dongbin. He then became their disciple and they passed on their Taoist lineage to him. Wang practiced their teachings diligently and became a well-known master. He ended up living in a compound built for him by his disciples that was known as "The Complete Realization," which then became the name of his school of Taoism.

Wang attempted to bring together the best elements of the three philosophical and spiritual teachings that dominated China at the time—Taoism, Buddhism, and Confucianism. From Confucianism he took the teachings on morality, emphasizing the need to do good deeds. From Buddhism he took the ideas of karma, simplicity, and the spontaneous enlightenment teachings of Chan (Zen). And from the Taoist tradition he took the ideas of spontaneity and existence in harmony with nature. Moving away from the more external aspects of these philosophies, such as elaborate ceremonies, charms, and intricate visualizations, he emphasized the internal aspects—self-cultivation through meditation and the alchemy.

Wang had many students but is renowned for seven disciples— six men and one woman—who are sometimes known as the Seven True Taoists of the North. These seven Taoist masters each had their own unique and colorful story. One was a drunk, one lived for a time in a brothel, one disfigured herself so she would be left alone, and each was known for possessing supernatural powers. These types of unusual, iconoclastic and irreverent personalities are typically associated with Taoism—a tradition that encourages its followers to find their own path to enlightenment.

Each of the seven masters expressed the Complete Reality teachings in their own way, creating seven different lineages:

Following Wang's death the seven disciples dispersed. One of them, Ch'iu Ch'ang-ch'un (Qiu Chuji), followed a quiet, ascetic life, living in caves and begging for food. He lived for several years in the Dragon Gate Cave, from which his sect draws its name. It was here that Ch'iu began to develop his teachings.

Later in his life he gained favor with the emperor and then with the conquering Mongol ruler, Genghis Khan, who honored him with the title Spirit Immortal. With this recognition and support the Complete Reality school grew very quickly. Ch'iu gained a large following, and over the years the Dragon Gate sect spread to many parts of China. At one time, the school became so popular that there was an expression that "the Dragon Gate Covers Half the Land." Ch'iu spent the last few years of his life in Beijing living at a Taoist temple now known as the White Cloud Temple (the most famous Taoist temple in China), and was buried there after his death. Since that time, the White Cloud temple has been the seat and headquarters for both the Complete Reality and Dragon Gate sects.

The Dragon Gate Taoism referred to in this book is part of a branch that took hold in Taiwan after the Communist takeover of mainland China forced all spiritual practitioners into hiding. In the relative freedom of Taiwan, the Dragon Gate practice continued to flourish and developed a unique system known as the Five Taoist Arts, which include:

- **Mountain**: a method of training to achieve physical and spiritual wholeness and longevity through proper diet, exercise, meditation, chi gung (qi gong, internal energy exercises), martial arts, and mantra.
- **Medical Science:** a method that combines Western medical practices where appropriate (in the Taoist tradition of absorbing what is useful) and traditional Chinese healing practices including acupuncture, herbal treatments and spiritual therapy (which addresses psycho-spiritual causes for illness) in order to achieve holistic healing and health maintenance.
- **Celestial Divination:** a method of revealing the life principles and laws governing human fate by observing micro and macrocosmic patterns as shown through a person's birth chart in combination with Book of Changes numerology.

- **Metamorphospection:** a method of observing the morphological (form and structure) characteristics in nature and people. Using methods such as feng shui, the metamorphospection method analyzes the external conditions of a person, building, or location.

- **Pu Divination:** a method of selecting optimal time and place for action by combining the time at which events are to take place, the time the divination is taking place, and the location and orientation of objects under consideration.

All of these Five Taoist Arts are used in combination in order to create as auspicious circumstances as possible for the Taoist practitioner to achieve their goals.

In summary, Dragon Gate Taoism offers a unique combination of philosophy, martial arts, meditation, magic, mysticism, and internal alchemy that makes this particular form of Taoism something truly extraordinary.

Taoist Alchemy

Nan Po asked: "How is it that you are old, Sir, but your complexion is like that of a child?"

Chuang Tzu responded: "I have become acquainted with the Tao."

—Chuang Tzu

Taoist alchemy dates back to the beginnings of Chinese history, thousands of years ago. Its goal was the attainment of spiritual and physical immortality. In ancient China, the pursuit of immortality on a physical or spiritual basis was an integral aspect of high culture. As Lao Tzu wrote: "He who dies and does not perish, has longevity."

There were several paths to immortality in the Taoist view, including:

- developing a form of consciousness that did not disintegrate after death
- giving birth to an immortal spiritual "baby"
- gradually transforming the physical body into an immortal body of light

The development of a form of consciousness that survives death is very similar to Buddhist ideas of enlightenment and involves the use of energy exercises to enable the consciousness to regain the state it was in before birth. Once a practitioner has achieved this state of being, their consciousness is able to leave the body and they are also able to retain their consciousness after death, thereby attaining a form of immortality.

Giving birth to a spiritual baby, or the "inner copulation" as it is often called, is a process in which the practitioner's energy develops to the point where the spirit and energy unite to form a spiritual baby, or a kind of second self that possesses the same consciousness but is not bound by physical laws or the material plane of reality. The spiritual entity is trained to be able to leave the physical body (which then appears lifeless) and return at will. After several years of successful practice the baby becomes an earthbound immortal and can exist apart from the body. The original consciousness is thus free from physical death because it is not dependent on the physical body for existence.

Transforming the physical body into an immortal body of light involves a process in which the spiritual body is combined with the physical body until the material form dissolves into a being composed of pure energy. This is also sometimes referred to as achieving the "rainbow body."

The Taoist focus on immortality also led to the development of numerous practices designed to promote health and longevity such as advanced breathing and energy exercises, including tai chi, as well as various dietary and lifestyle regimes. These, in turn, were incorporated into the alchemy.

Taoist alchemy can be separated into two major branches: external and internal. The external alchemy sought physical immortality through the ingestion of an elixir, often concocted from toxic substances. The internal alchemy created the elixir internally though the preservation and cultivation of the vital essences of the body.

Although there are major differences between the two types of practice, they have a number of technical terms in common. In fact, many formulas for the internal, "golden elixir" alchemy disguise instructions by substituting physical substances for counterparts within the human body. For example, lead and mercury represent vitality and spirit. It is possible that the external alchemy is actually a degeneration of the internal branch caused by the literal interpretation of the metaphorical terminology that was used to keep the work secret.

The internal alchemy described in this book involves using a set of advanced exercises, meditations, visualizations, and, if appropriate, sexual yoga practices to turn your physical reproductive life force into chi, or energy. The energy is then further refined until it becomes spirit. And finally, over time you learn to unify your spirit with the Tao, or all that is.

This formula is described as follows: "Through compounding reproductive energy (ching), the internal energy (chi) is transformed; through compounding the internal energy, the spirit (shen) is transformed." Thus, ching, chi, and shen are the fundamental elements in the process of meditative breathing.

THE TAOIST ALCHEMICAL FORMULA

1. Reproductive (or sexual) energy is turned into chi (vital internal energy).
2. Chi is further refined into spirit (consciousness).
3. Spirit is transformed into void, or the potentiality of everything.
4. Once in the void, consciousness can merge with the Tao (the supreme way of nature, or all that is).

This formula can be considered the highest level of Dragon Gate energy practices.

Each of the precious substances used in the alchemy has a twofold nature and functions on an individual level in humans and on a cosmic level within the universe.

Ching (jing), which is also translated as essence, in its material form is manifested as our reproductive (and sexual) fluids. It represents the tremendous sexual energy within people that maintains the vitality of the human body and has the power to create new life. On a universal level, ching is the life energy of heaven and earth that causes the light of the sun and moon and growth and fertility in nature.

Chi (qi) is translated as vital, internal energy (it is also sometimes translated as breath). It is of paramount importance in Taoist practice because it is our source of energy, created by the refinement of the ching and cultivated by breathing techniques, exercises, and sexual yoga. Taoist meditation focuses on breathing as smoothly and naturally as an infant in keeping with Taoist tradition.

Lao Tzu wrote: "When one gives undivided attention to the (vital) breath, and brings it to the utmost degree of pliancy, he can become as a tender babe." In the Inner Elixir school this was often referred to as embryonic breathing. On a universal level chi is the energy behind heaven and earth that provides the impetus for perpetual change.

Shen, or spirit, refers to our spiritual consciousness. In the alchemical process, we use the chi, our energy, to activate our spiritual consciousness and free it from the potentially limiting effects of our normal physical reality and day-to-day mental processes. The refinement of spirit in turn leads to the attainment of Tao, or union.

The union with Tao also relates to the mental awakening that occurs when you have successfully practiced the alchemy. The essential idea is that before birth you have a pristine, untarnished state of enlightened consciousness without a false idea of self or other. After birth, you learn to perceive in terms of the language and norms imposed by your culture. This socialization process obscures the original, innate purity of perception. By relaxing the mind into its natural state, the Dragon Gate practitioner regains his original mind.

Spiritual awakening cannot occur until a free flow of energy has been achieved by greatly increasing the amount of chi circulating throughout the body. The physical process that unites the body and mind and develops and causes the chi to circulate freely throughout the energy centers of the body, is the source of all life—breathing.

The Dragon Gate breathing and meditation exercises described throughout this book is a very safe, effective, and quick method of developing and circulating the tremendous energy potential we all have. Through its emphasis on natural, unforced breathing, Dragon Gate is also a means of balancing the flow of chi and returning the mind to its original consciousness at the body's own pace and in harmony with the energy forces of nature.

Understanding the Tao is like trying to cage the wind.

—Siji Tzu

Universal Harmonization Practice

We conclude this chapter with a simple but powerful alchemical exercise designed to activate your energy centers and prepare you for the exercises that follow in the rest of the book.

Find a comfortable place to lie down on your back. This can be inside or outside, but you should make sure that you can lie comfortably for a period of time and that there are no major distractions such as noise, weather, etc. that could disturb you. It's a good idea to turn off the phone and anything else that may disturb your practice.

Make sure you are wearing something loose and comfortable. Also, you will need to have bare feet for this exercise.

1. Lie down.
2. Close your eyes, relax, and take 3 very deep breaths, filling and emptying your lungs completely each time.
3. Begin by activating the energy points on the bottom of your feet. This point, referred to as the "bubbling spring well" is the Chinese acupuncture point, Kidney 1, which is the beginning of the water channel. It is located on the bottom of the foot, beneath the arch, in the depression in the center of the sole. This point is of great significance in Taoist practice since it is our connection with the earth. To activate these points imagine each one as a spiral vortex of energy.
4. Once you clearly sense the bubbling spring well energy point, activate the points in the center of your palms. To activate these points imagine each one as a spiral vortex of energy.
5. Now you will activate each of the major energy centers along the spinal column. The activation uses the seven colors of the visible spectrum—the rainbow—to activate the seven major energy centers. These colors can easily be remembered with the old high school mnemonic device of "Roy G. Biv" (red, orange, yellow, green, blue, indigo, violet).
6. Become aware of the energy center at the base of the spine. Now visualize a red light shining from that point.
7. Become aware of the energy center at your navel. Now visualize an orange light shining from that point.
8. Become aware of the energy center at your solar plexus. Now visualize a yellow light shining from that point.

9. Become aware of the energy center at your heart (in the center of your chest). Now visualize a green light shining from that point.

10. Become aware of the energy center at the throat. Now visualize a blue light shining from that point.

11. Become aware of the energy center at the base of the nose directly between your two eyes. Now visualize an indigo (bluish-purple) light shining from that point.

12. Become aware of the energy center at the top of your head. Now visualize a violet light shining from that point.

13. Now simply lie for a few moments with each of your energy centers activated and radiating the rainbow spectrum of light.

You can spend as much time as you wish focusing on each energy center, but you should spend a minimum of 1 minute. With practice you will find that you can obtain excellent energy development and rejuvenation from this exercise within a few minutes, but you may also find this an extremely worthwhile form of meditation to practice for longer periods of time.

This method of meditation may also be used prior to going to sleep at night or before a nap and can help the practice of dream yoga (as detailed in Chapter 6, "Taoist Shamanism and Dream Yoga").

Second Gate:
The Foundations of Health

DRAGON GATE FOUNDATION PRACTICES FOR HEALTH

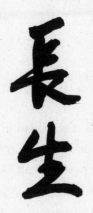

Longevity

When man is born he is tender and soft. At death he is stiff and hard. All things, the grass as well as the trees, are tender and supple while alive. When dead they are withered and dried. Therefore, the stiff and hard are companions of death. The tender and soft are companions of life.

—LAO TZU

Please take a moment now before you begin this chapter to practice this brief and simple exercise. It will help you to maximize your enjoyment of the chapter.

Find a mirror where you can look at yourself comfortably (without having to hold the mirror). Now look at yourself in the mirror and without breaking your gaze repeat the following 3 times:

"I love myself and I always will."

Now you are ready to begin.

Health Is Wealth

The quality of your life is determined in large part by the quality of your health. Good health is the foundation that enables you to succeed in life and in the pursuit of all your goals—including spiritual enlightenment—by having the mental clarity to find what works for you, the energy to achieve your objectives, and the stamina to follow your path to its destination. Additionally, most physical ailments and psychological problems can be greatly alleviated or completely eliminated through proper diet, exercise, and lifestyle.

That is why the Dragon Gate school of Taoism has evolved a complete system of chi-gung, or qi gong, breathing and energy development exercises, Taoist yoga and martial arts designed to provide practitioners with excellent health, fitness, and mental acuity.

This chapter covers the foundation Dragon Gate practices for health, including the six keys to a healthy life.

Six Keys to a Healthy Life

Health is the greatest possession.

—LAO TZU

I'm sure you've heard the old sayings "health is wealth" and "if you have your health, you have everything." Unfortunately, this often becomes most obvious to people when they are sick or injured. There is no doubt that it is far more difficult to follow any path when your body or your mind ails you. On a physical level, when you are ill or injured, you are more likely to compound those illnesses and injuries, while simultaneously finding it more difficult to generate the energy required to pull yourself out of the negative situation. On a mental level, when you are healthy, you can deal with life's difficult situations without getting stressed out or depressed and you have more energy to participate in activities that reaffirm your enjoyment of life.

In keeping with the Taoist approach, the path to excellent health does not require elaborate rituals, exercises, or activities. There are a number of basic things you can do to attain and maintain generally excellent physical and mental health, vitality, and energy. What is required is a return to the natural patterns associated with good health. To this end there is a simple program based on six keys associated with breathing, drinking, eating, sleeping, exercising, and meditating. These six keys are derived from an analysis of the way humans live. In other words, what is required for us to live and also what can we truly not live well without.

The following six keys to a healthy, happy life are also a checklist you can look to any time you are feeling ill or down. Just go over the list and see how you're doing. If you find that one or more of these six keys is not being adequately taken care of in your life, now is the time to start. As Lao Tzu wrote: "A journey of a thousand miles begins with a single step."

So here are the six keys, in order of importance.

First Key: Breathe Like a Taoist

Breathing is the first key. Why? Because it is the single most important action you take in life. If you stop breathing you will die within minutes. The average person can hold their breath for only a minute or two before passing out and then dying if air is not restored. The world record for holding the breath (unassisted) is eight minutes, eight seconds for men and six minutes, six seconds for women, and close to thirteen minutes with assistance (for example, pre-breathing 100 percent oxygen).

Air is undoubtedly the single most important thing we take into our bodies. That is obvious, but despite its importance to our lives, as a general rule, people are not taught how to breathe it. It's something we do so naturally that we take it for granted and unless you're a woman taking a Lamaze class during pregnancy or someone who has chosen to focus on breathing as part of a sport, or spiritual practice, chances are you don't think much about it. But as with any activity there are better and worse ways to breathe.

Taoists often compare proper breathing to the way a baby breathes. Lao Tzu, in the *Tao Te Ching* wrote: "The sage maintains harmony by breathing like a sleeping babe." We all started in the womb breathing from our navel. If you watch infants you will see that their stomachs expand and contract with their breathing. This is because they are breathing from their abdomens, as they did when they were connected to their mothers through the umbilical cord. That is why the navel—otherwise known as the dantian (t'an-tien)—is considered the key energy center in Taoist physiognomy. As an adult, you should be doing the same thing—that is, breathing from the abdomen.

Chuang Tzu, after Lao Tzu the second most famous Taoist sage wrote: "The true Man of ancient times slept without dreaming and woke without care; he ate without savoring and his breath came from deep inside. The true man breathes with his heels; the mass of men breathe with their throats. Crushed and bound down, they gasp out their words as though they are retching. Deep in their passions and desires they are shallow in the workings of Heaven." What this refers to is that most people take very shallow breaths, providing their body with a minimal amount of oxygen, while the best breathing is very deep.

If your breathing is shallow and weak you are starving your body of the oxygen that it needs to run. Oxygen is at the heart of every process in the human body. So learn how to do deep breathing (if you don't already know) and learn how to breathe from your abdomen. If you are feeling low, a few minutes of deep breathing will work wonders.

It is also important to note that from the Taoist perspective, breathing is an essential part of how one cultivates the chi, or life energy force (more on this in the next chapter). Proper breathing is the root of all spiritual practices, and learning how to do it correctly is of prime importance.

☯ Dragon Gate Basic Breathing Method

(Chapter 3, "Breathing and the Development of Chi," goes into greater depth on Dragon Gate methods of breathing and provides several exercises. In addition there are many other breathing exercises throughout this book. For a complete listing check the exercise index at the beginning of this book.)

The following basic breathing exercise is recommended as a way to begin training in correct Dragon Gate breathing methods.

1. Find a comfortable place to lie down. Make sure that there are no major distractions such as noise, weather, etc.

2. Make sure that you have nothing binding on your body, so remove your shoes and if you are wearing a belt, undo it (it's also a good idea to loosen your pants or skirt).

3. Allow your body to relax completely. It is often helpful to think of yourself floating down a stream.

4. Inhale slowly, steadily and deeply to your abdomen, focusing on your navel. As you inhale relax your entire body and especially your abdomen to allow your lungs to expand to their full capacity.

5. Exhale slowly and steadily, making sure to completely empty all the air in your lungs.

6. Repeat 9 times. You can practice this exercise more or fewer times depending on how you feel.

Second Key: Drink Enough Water

Drinking enough water is the second key. Why? After air, the body's second greatest need is water. People will die of thirst within a matter of days and virtually no one can last longer than a week without it. It makes sense, considering that between 45 and 75 percent of the weight of a human body is from water. Infants have the highest concentration at 75 percent, while about 60 percent of the weight of the average man and about 55 percent of that of the average woman is water.

Water is your most essential nutrient. Every system in your body depends on it. So it stands to reason that drinking an adequate amount of water is an extremely important element of good health.

Not coincidentally, drinking enough good, clean water is probably the single easiest and most powerful thing you can do to improve your health. Alarmingly, a majority of Americans are chronically dehydrated. Studies have associated dehydration with fatigue, joint pain, mental strain, and other common ailments. In fact, dehydration is the number one cause of headaches and heartburn.

☯ Why is drinking water good for you?

- Water helps keep our bodies clean by moving waste out of our bodies through the breath, sweat, and urine. It also flushes toxins from the body.
- Studies have shown that drinking enough water decreases the risk of colon, bladder, urinary tract, and breast cancer.
- Water helps people attain and maintain a healthy weight. It does this by suppressing the appetite, aiding in digestion and the absorption of nutrients, preventing constipation, and helping the body to metabolize fat.
- Water helps eliminate mental fatigue, impaired concentration, and foggy short-term memory.

- Water cushions and lubricates your joints and muscles. It can also help reduce cramping and fatigue during workouts.
- Water supports the body's lymphatic system, which produces antibodies and carries waste fluids from the cells.

☯ *How much water should you drink?*

When it comes to the amount of water you should drink, there are countless variations on the advice given. There is a common recommendation of eight 8-ounce glasses per day. But there is no single formula that fits all people in all situations. A person's height, weight, and level of activity factor into the equation, as does the time of year and location. If you're in the desert in summer, you're going to need a lot more water than during the fall in a cold, damp place, and a large person who works out heavily will require a lot more water than a small, sedentary one.

The Taoist approach would be to drink when you are thirsty. However, that also requires the sensitivity to know when your body is thirsty and for many people the thirst mechanism is so weak that it is often mistaken for hunger. But if you work on it, you can become more aware of your thirst mechanism.

A couple of guidelines you can follow are: drink throughout the day, because unless you're exercising, your body can only process a limited amount of water at a time—about 8 ounces per hour. Also, your urine should be colorless or light yellow (unless you're eating food or vitamins that change your urine color).

☯ *What should you drink?*

Many people drink caffeinated drinks (such as coffee or sodas) all day. Caffeine is a diuretic and actually works to remove water from your body. Juice and sodas contain a lot of sugar, which is not good for you, and high fructose corn syrup, which is much worse. Diet sodas are bad for you on many levels and should be avoided. Aside from the fact that diet sodas contain two of the most harmful ingredients in our food supply (aspartame and Splenda), numerous studies have shown that these ingredients actually cause people to gain weight. Even though diet drinks have no calories, they actually stimulate your appetite and cause a powerful craving for carbohydrates. Other research suggests that artificial sweeteners also stimulate fat storage.

So you should get your liquid in the form of water and water-rich fruits and vegetables. But you should think twice before drinking unfiltered tap water. One major reason is the presence of chlorine, which is a biocide added to the water supply to keep it free of harmful bacteria. While chlorine keeps us from getting cholera and other waterborne diseases, the chlorine in your tap water can interact with organic matter in aging pipes and can produce several known carcinogens. Because of this, some cities are already implementing alternative water treatments and replacing chlorine with a chemical substitute called chloramine (a blend of chlorine and ammonia). Unfortunately, chloramine has been linked to the production of by-products that are more toxic than those produced by chlorine. What's worse, the toxic effects of these by-products have not been studied and scientists simply don't know what kind of damage they can cause.

You can inexpensively neutralize the chlorine in tap water by adding a pinch of vitamin C. But the best way to remove chlorine and chloramine is to filter the water using a good filtration system. Most home and portable water filtering units remove organic and inorganic compounds—including lead and other metals, chlorine, chloramine, trihalomethanes, and radon gas.

Distillation is another method for creating pure H_2O. Just be aware that there are studies that indicate there are potential problems with distilled water—namely that the absence of minerals will cause them to be leeched from the body. So if you choose to drink distilled water, you will want to add minerals (which you can purchase at most health food stores) back to the water.

DRAGON GATE WATER EXERCISE

The Dragon Gate system believes that you can turn any activity into a spiritual practice. With that in mind, ancient masters developed numerous simple techniques that you can incorporate into your daily life. The Dragon Gate glass of water exercise is one such method. It is not something you need to do each time you drink water, but you may find it very useful to incorporate it into your cupboard of Dragon Gate techniques.

- When you go to get a drink of water, pause for a moment before filling your glass and take a deep breath to your navel.
- Focus your mind on a goal that you desire. It can be anything, from finishing an important task to eliminating a headache to feeling blissful.
- Holding your goal in mind, fill your glass with water.
- Focus your attention on the full glass and feel the energy from your intention energizing the water and attuning it to your goal.
- Drink all the water.

Third Key: Eat Well

Eating is the third key. Why? If you stop eating you'll die within weeks. Your body needs food for energy, regeneration, healing, and so on. Check what you're eating. If you need to, make a list of what you eat. Get rid of the garbage and put in the healthy, nutrient-filled foods that you know are good for you. If you're feeling low, after ensuring that you are drinking enough water, make sure you are eating a balanced and healthy diet.

Former surgeon general C. Everett Koop has said that 70 percent of all Americans are dying from diseases that are directly tied to their eating habits. Perhaps the simplest recommendation for healthy eating is to avoid sugar and its even more evil relative, high fructose corn syrup, which is arguably the single worst ingredient in most processed foods you purchase today. These sweeteners are associated with a plethora of health problems including the depletion of minerals and other nutrients in the body, immune depression, diabetes, and cancer—just to name a few. Many foods (especially processed snack foods) have tons of sugar. (Learn to read the labels on the food you buy. It can be very enlightening.)

So what should you eat? Michael Pollan, the author of *The Omnivore's Dilemma,* put it succinctly: "Eat food. Not too much. Mostly plants." His humorous food haiku is actually very much in line with the Taoist perspective, which is to eat wholesome foods and only when you are truly hungry. For many people, however, hunger is an omnipresent feeling. Two of the best things for reducing hunger are drinking plenty of water and exercising (two of the other six keys).

As a general recommendation, you should eat whole (unprocessed) foods with an emphasis on fruits, vegetables, seeds, nuts, and legumes. Diets that are primarily vegetarian based have been shown to provide numerous health benefits, including improved cardiovascular function, reduced weight, lower incidences of cancer, and longer lifespan. (If you are a vegetarian you need to ensure that you are getting a full, balanced diet with plenty of protein.) Whenever possible try to eat food that is organic because it does not have pesticides, preservatives, or hormones, all of which are bad for you. (Additional recommendations on healthy foods can be found in Chapter 4, "Cultivating the Mind.")

If you look around America you might think what people really need to do is stop eating; obesity is a national epidemic. But the solution isn't to stop eating; the solution is to eat correctly and combine it with a healthy lifestyle that includes exercise.

Here are several simple ways to lose weight and keep it off:

- Eat breakfast. Several studies have shown that not eating breakfast significantly increases your risk of obesity.
- Eat a healthy snack in the afternoon.
- Drink a little water with every meal. It will help you feel full.
- Do not eat in front of the TV. This leads to mindless eating, which is a major contributor to obesity.
- Plan your meals.
- Eat high protein and low-glycemic foods (the glycemic index is a measure of the effects of carbohydrates on blood sugar levels).
- Begin a regular and effective exercise program.

Dragon Gate Food Exercise

The Dragon Gate food exercise is very similar to the water exercise outlined above. Like the water exercise, the food exercise is not something you need to do each time you eat. It is for special instances when you feel it is warranted.

1. Before you begin a meal, pause for a moment, sit down, and take a deep breath to your navel.
2. Focus your mind on a goal that you desire.
3. Speaking aloud or silently (depending on the situation) say to yourself, "May this meal provide me with the energy to pursue the Tao and fulfill all my dreams."
4. Begin eating.

Fourth Key: Sleep Well

The fourth key is sleeping. Why? If you stop sleeping you'll experience serious mental problems, often within days. The body needs its sleep cycle and REM state to rest, recuperate, regenerate, and so on. According to the National Sleep Foundation nearly two-thirds of American adults do not get the nightly eight hours of sleep recommended for good health and optimum performance. Sleep problems include difficulty falling asleep, waking up in the night, feeling unrefreshed upon rising, and sleep apnea. Moreover, the effects of sleep deprivation are cumulative. And if you are not sleeping well, you have a problem that goes beyond feeling stressed, angry, sad, and mentally exhausted.

As you might expect, drowsiness causes accidents—more than

100,000 a year in North America alone. And lack of sleep has been shown to reduce immune function and aggravate conditions including hypertension, diabetes, and obesity. Even more worrisome, statistics show that how long you live is related to the amount of sleep you obtain on average per night. Mortality rates are lowest for people who report sleeping seven to nine hours a night.

Here are a number of suggestions to improve your sleeping if you are having problems:

- Avoid sleeping pills or any other supplement designed to induce drowsiness. These are for emergencies only.
- Avoid naps during the day (unless they are part of your normal sleep schedule).
- Spend time in the sun every day.
- Do some aerobic exercise during the day.
- Eliminate sugar and lower your overall intake of carbohydrates.
- Reduce or eliminate caffeine and other stimulants and avoid taking them later in the day.

You should, of course, do your best to follow the other five keys to a healthy life outlined in this chapter. If you follow the six keys listed here it will help you to have a good night's sleep.

Dragon Gate Easy Sleeping Exercise

The following method can be used to help you fall asleep if you are having difficulties.

1. Before going to sleep do your best to ensure that your sleeping environment is quiet, dark, peaceful, and comfortable. Once the room is prepared, lie down in your bed and make yourself as comfortable as you can by positioning your body and pillows and blankets in the optimal position. Make sure that you have nothing binding on your body.

2. Allow your body to relax completely. It is often helpful to think of yourself floating down a stream.

3. Take 3 very deep breaths, inhaling slowly, steadily, and deeply to your abdomen, while focusing on your navel, and then exhaling slowly and steadily.

4. Now, in your mind's eye, visualize a bright, full moon. On the face of the moon see the number 9 appear. Now see a soft and fluffy cloud pass over the moon and the number 9 disappears. Then the number 8 fades in on the moon. The clouds then float over the moon and the number 8 disappears.

5. Repeat this process counting down slowly and evenly for 7, 6, 5, 4, 3, 2, 1, and 0.

6. Once you have reached 0, begin the process again at 9 and continue until you fall asleep. You will find that the more you use the exercise the faster it will work.

Fifth Key: Exercise Regularly

Regular exercise is an essential part of keeping your mind and body healthy. As the Taoist expression goes, "A working hinge has no rust." If you stop exercising you won't die, but you will certainly feel the negative consequences. Countless studies have shown the enormous benefits to be had from exercise, including:

- Improving your mood
- Combating chronic disease
- Managing your appetite and weight and improving your appearance
- Strengthening your heart and lungs
- Promoting better sleep and better sex
- Preserving and enhancing mental functions

If you exercise regularly you can forestall many illnesses and injuries. The key areas (in order of importance are): a) agility, so stretch regularly; b) strength, so do body weight calisthenics and/or some weight training regularly; and c) cardiovascular, so do something that gets your heart beating and your lungs pumping on a regular basis (but avoid high-stress, high-impact exercises). The most important thing with exercise is doing something every day. Ten minutes a day is much better than 70 minutes done once a week. This is what makes the difference between a healthy old age and a decrepit old age. As a guideline, exercising at least 30 minutes at least 4 times per week is the minimum.

Before doing the following exercises, ensure that you are wearing loose-fitting and comfortable exercise clothes and good exercise shoes.

DRAGON GATE AGILITY EXERCISE: THE DRAGON REACHES FOR THE PEARL

1. Find a place where you can elevate your leg to a comfortable height. A railing, countertop, tabletop, or any other stable surface will do. The heel of the elevated leg should be no less

than knee height and no more than slightly above waist height. It is best to have the elevated leg at just above waist height if you are comfortable in that position. Make sure the ground or floor is flat and not slippery.

2. Raise your left leg and place it on the platform you will be using to elevate your leg. Make sure the left (elevated) leg is straight. Keep the right leg (the one you are standing on) straight, but do not lock the right knee. If you have trouble balancing yourself, stand where you can place one hand on a railing, wall, or other support.

3. Keeping your body square so that your chest is facing your left foot, place the palm of your left hand facing up at your waist.

4. Breathe in. Now, exhaling slowly in sync with the movement, slowly extend your left hand toward the toes of your left (elevated) foot and as you extend your hand turn your palm over very slowly so that by the end of the extension your left palm is facing down. Extend your left arm as far as is comfortable without strain. Remember to do the extension very slowly. The slower you can do it, the better. Taking 5 seconds to complete the extension is a minimum, but 10 seconds is ideal.

5. Slowly retract your left hand back toward your waist (where it began the extension). As you bring your hand back, turn your palm over very slowly so that by the time it is back by your waist, your left palm is facing up once again. Remember to do the retraction very slowly. The slower you can do it, the better. Taking 5 seconds to complete the retraction is a minimum, but 10 seconds is ideal.

6. Repeat this extension/retraction process 9 times.

7. Now switch legs and do the same thing with your right foot
   elevated and extending/retracting your right palm. Remember to breathe out as you extend your palm and breathe in
   as you retract your palm.

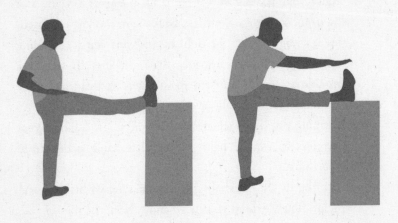

DRAGON GATE BASIC STRENGTH EXERCISE:
HOLD THE MOON AND REACH FOR THE SUN

Dragon Gate strength exercises are rooted in Chinese martial arts.
Therefore your strength is built from the bottom up—unlike many
Western traditions that focus much more on the upper body. The
Chinese martial arts tradition calls your legs and the stances you
hold with them your "horse," since it is what moves you where
you want to go. There are many different body-weight and weighted
exercises that you can practice, but it is best to develop the strength
in your legs first. The leg muscles are large and when they are
properly developed they can help you in all your workouts.

1. Find a flat, level surface. Stand with your feet shoulder-
   width apart, hands at your sides, looking straight ahead.

(You can wear sneakers or stand barefoot if you are very comfortable that way.)

2. Breathe in slowly. Then, exhaling slowly in sync with the movement, very slowly bend your knees. Keep your fingers pointed to the ground as you lower your body. It is very important to keep your back straight throughout the exercise and to move very slowly. You also want to synchronize your breathing and the movement of your arms and legs according to the instructions.

3. Go as low as you feel comfortable. For most people this means going no lower than the point where your thighs are parallel to the ground. If you are in excellent health and your knees are fine, you can go all the way down, but you are strongly urged to build up to this over time. As you lower your body, bring your hands together in front of you, palms up, with your fingertips almost touching. It should feel as though you are holding a large beach ball.

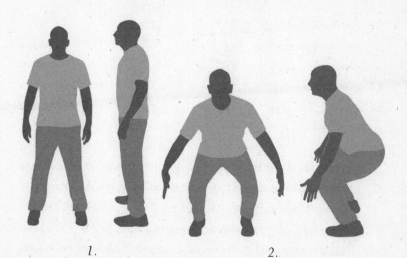

1.   2.

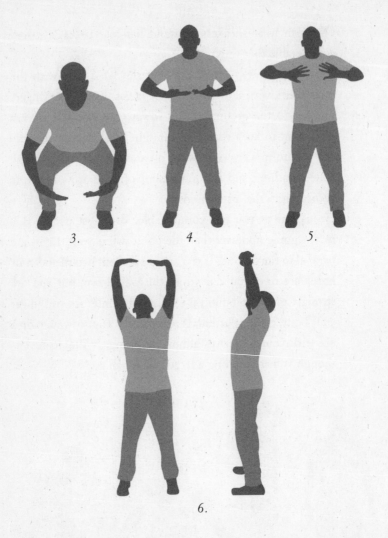

3.   4.   5.

6.

4. Now, inhaling slowly in sync with the movement, stand back up so that you return to your starting position. As you return to the original position slowly raise your palms, the finger-tips should be almost touching. Once your palms reach your solar plexus level, they should turn over so that the palms are

facing up. Then, exhaling slowly in sync with the movement, continue to straighten your legs (do not lock your knees) and push your palms straight up toward the sky.

5. Now, exhaling slowly in sync with the movement, lower your palms back to your sides and back to the starting position.

6. Repeat this exercise for a total of 9 times.

DRAGON GATE STAMINA EXERCISE: DRAGON WALKING

1. Find a flat and level place to practice where there is room for a circle with a diameter of 10 to 15 feet. (You can wear sneakers or go barefoot if you are very comfortable that way and there is nothing on the ground that would hurt your feet.)

2. Place an object in the middle of the circle (this can be anything from a small stick to a tennis ball—it is just used to mark the center of the circle).

3. Stand on the edge of the circle with your body in line with the circle (perpendicular to the center).

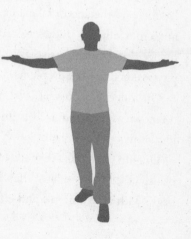

4. Extend your arms to the sides so that your palms face up and your arms are in line with your body and parallel to the ground. Your palms should be at shoulder height.

5. Begin walking around the circle. Start your walk slowly and with each rotation increase the speed so that by the last rotation you are walking as quickly as you can while maintaining complete stability.

6. Do 9 rotations of the circle. Then stop. Face the center of the circle and breathe deeply 9 times.

7. Now turn your body in the opposite direction and do the same exercise in the other direction.

Sixth Key: Meditate Regularly

Meditation represents the sixth and final key to physical health and happiness. It is, of course, the mental key. Each of us needs some time of quiet contemplation on a regular basis to detach from the hustle and bustle of life, to silence the internal dialogue that can keep us stuck in a certain way of viewing the world, and to put the petty problems that gnaw at us into perspective. Regular meditators typically report feeling happier, more peaceful, and more present. But beyond the anecdotal evidence, meditation has been shown in numerous clinical studies to reduce stress, foster physical health, reduce chronic pain, assist with sleeping, and help with many other physical and mental problems.

On a deeper, spiritual level, meditation is a doorway into the unknown aspects of ourselves, and it can help us to unravel the mystery of who we really are.

Dragon Gate has a very advanced system of meditation that will be discussed more in later chapters, however, for now it is useful to begin with a very simple and effective meditation exercise.

DRAGON GATE SITTING MEDITATION: THE DRAGON RESTS

Sitting meditation is the root form of meditation. It is extremely simple to do and all you need is a chair.

Find a quiet, peaceful place to practice. Make sure that there are no major distractions such as noise, weather, etc. Remember to stay calm and relaxed throughout the whole meditation.

1. Make sure that you have nothing binding on your body, so if you are wearing a belt, undo it (it's also a good idea to loosen your pants or skirt).

2. Set a timer for 5 minutes. You can increase the amount of time you spend meditating, but we recommend starting with 5 minutes and then increasing it by 2 to 5 minute intervals as you feel inclined. We recommend using a timer with a soft, enjoyable alarm (many cell phones now have alarms where you can select the tone and volume you wish) that you place in another room, so you can faintly hear it, but so that it is not disturbing when it goes off. It's a very doable amount of time. If you are more comfortable meditating without a timer, feel free to do so. A timer allows you to forget about how long you are sitting, but some people find it more relaxing to meditate without it.

3. Sit on the edge of a solid, armless chair that doesn't move (no wheels or swivel) with your buttocks and legs supporting your weight. At the ideal height your hips should be slightly above your knees. It is fine to place a small cushion on the chair to give yourself a small elevation. Your feet

should be firmly placed on the floor, shoulder width apart, knees bent at close to a 90-degree angle. The shoulders and elbows should be kept down throughout the meditation. Rest the hands, palms down, on the knees. The back should be straight at the waist, but slightly rounded at the shoulder and neck.

4. Allow your body to relax completely. It is often helpful to think of yourself floating down a stream.

5. Look straight ahead, chin parallel to the ground throughout the meditation (even when your eyes are closed).

6. Close your eyes.

7. Visualize a beautiful scene. This can be any scene that you find peaceful and attractive including a beach, a forest, a mountaintop, or any other location that you find relaxing. If you have trouble visualizing a scene, don't worry about it. The meditation works fine without a visualization. This is only meant to assist you in your practice.

8. Throughout the meditation, inhale slowly, steadily and deeply to your abdomen, focusing on your navel.

9. When your meditation is done, rub your hands briskly for a few seconds until you feel heat in your palms. Then rub your

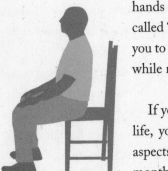

hands on your face, head, and body. This is called "bathing in the chi" and is a way for you to spread the energy you have gathered while meditating around your body.

If you follow these six keys to a healthy life, you will notice improvements in all aspects of your life usually in less than a month and sometimes much faster. Regular practice of these methods will ensure a higher state of mental, physical, and spiritual well-being.

In conclusion, we would like to note that the six keys presented in this chapter are designed to assist you in achieving a basic level of health and vitality that will enable you to move forward in your spiritual path and assist you in finding happiness. But it is also very important to remember that all health—mental and physical—is predicated on the requirement that you love yourself—which is why the chapter began with an exercise designed to promote self-love. This is not the same thing as being self-absorbed, conceited, or egotistical. Quite the contrary, self-love, from a Taoist perspective, refers to achieving a level of appreciation and enjoyment for the gifts you have and forgiveness for the areas where you find yourself falling short of your expectations. So the six keys are also designed to help you to love yourself more as you proceed on the path to health.

Third Gate: Breathing and the Development of Chi

DRAGON GATE BREATHING EXERCISES

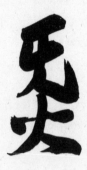

Chi

Breathing control gives man strength, vitality, inspiration, and magic powers.

—CHUANG TZU

Please take a moment now before you begin this chapter to practice this brief and simple exercise. It will help you to maximize your enjoyment of the chapter.

Find a comfortable place to sit or lie down. Close your eyes. Simply become aware of your breathing for a minute or two.

Now you are ready to begin.

The Root Exercise

Improper breathing is a common cause of ill health. If I had to limit my advice on healthier living to just one tip, it would be simply to learn how to breathe correctly. There's no single more powerful—or more simple—daily practice to further your health and well-being than breathwork.

—ANDREW WEIL, M.D.

It may seem obvious, but breathing is the single most important physical activity that you engage in. If you stop breathing for just a few minutes, you will cease to exist. This is the core reason that breathing is the root exercise in all Taoist practice and enormous emphasis is placed on learning and then practicing correct breathing until it becomes natural. If there is one lesson you can take away from this book, it will be how to be a better breather. It can make a huge difference on every level of your life—physical, mental, energetic and spiritual.

Breathing correctly is also the single most important key to developing your chi, or life energy, which is used for physical, mental, and spiritual advancement (more on this later). Taoists, known throughout China for their amazing longevity, have spent centuries developing a very advanced system of breathing exercises. Fortunately, while the philosophy behind the exercises is complex, many of the techniques are quite simple and easy to do, and the results can be felt within just a few weeks of practice.

The concept of the trinity of Heaven, Earth, and Man has influenced the majority of Chinese philosophical thought, as have the ideas of yin and yang and the five elements. Man is viewed as a microcosmic universe, and Taoists attempt to achieve a harmony of body and mind through breathing exercises.

On a physical level, when we breathe in, we provide our bodies with oxygen, which is our most important nutrient. (Here on earth, oxygen makes up about 21 percent of the gas in air.) Our bodies need oxygen in order to synthesize the chemical ATP (adenosine triphosphate), which provides our cells with most of the energy they require to function.

First, let's briefly review how we physically breathe.

- Muscles expand the chest cavity and air enters the body. (This is why the way you breathe can greatly affect the amount of air that you are inhaling.) The air is warmed, moistened, and cleaned by the upper airways before entering the lungs. Once in the lungs, the air travels through smaller and smaller tube-like structures until it reaches tiny air sacs, known as alveoli.
- Tiny blood vessels called capillaries carry our blood past the air sacs. The blood then picks up oxygen.
- Oxygenated blood rushes from the capillaries in the lungs through progressively larger blood vessels until it returns to the left side of the heart and is pumped throughout the body.
- The mitochondria in your cells, sometimes referred to as the cells' power plant, use oxygen to create most of the energy that powers our cells.
- The waste product in this respiratory process is carbon dioxide (CO_2), which is then expelled from the body when you exhale. This is the other half of the breathing equation, because not only are you inhaling a primary source of energy, but you are exhaling waste.

All chronic pain, suffering, and diseases are caused from
a lack of oxygen at the cell level.

—ARTHUR C. GUYTON, M.D.,
Textbook of Medical Physiology

Research has shown that lack of oxygen is a major cause of a
wide variety of problems, including everything from poor sleeping and reduced mental acuity to diminished immune function,
heart disease, stroke, and even cancer. It is important to note that
the brain requires more oxygen than any other organ. Though it
constitutes only 2 percent of the weight of the body, the brain con-
sumes about 20 percent of the body's total energy (at rest). The
mental consequences for insufficient oxygen are apparent and include irritability, an inability to think clearly, a decrease in sense
acuity, and memory loss.

The benefits of Taoist breathing include:

- Improved health and well-being
- Increased energy and vitality
- The efficient removal of toxins from the body
- Better digestion
- Superior mental functioning
- Stronger lungs
- Reduced strain on the heart (it doesn't have to work as hard
  to distribute the same amount of oxygen)
- Reduced mental and physical stress (the mind and body will
  be functioning on an optimal level)
- Improved sleeping

So, clearly, breathing correctly, in a manner designed to bring as much oxygen into the body as possible is essential to optimal health and well being. In China, *The Yellow Emperor's Classic of Internal Medicine* is considered to be the foundation of all traditional Chinese medicine. First written more than two thousand years ago, the book notes that people can remain healthy by "practicing deep breathing to allow the smooth flow of the chi throughout the body." Another book, entitled *Guangzi* (written approximately 300 B.C.) points out: "The practice of breathing will help improve the function of the eyes and ears and the general fitness of the four limbs, and this will in turn accumulate abundant energy and vigor in the body."

Proper breathing in a relaxed state increases awareness because of the increased oxygen flow to the brain and throughout the body. Taoists realized the vital importance of an adequate oxygen supply thousands of years ago and so they created and perfected numerous breathing techniques.

Breathing nourishes youthfulness.

—*The Jade Emperor's Mind Seal Classic*

For inspiration on proper breathing methods, the Taoists looked to the way babies breathe. If you have ever watched babies closely then perhaps you've noticed that their entire bodies expand and contract as they breathe. It looks as though they are using their entire bodies to breathe. Now take a look at most adults and if you watch closely you will see that their breathing has become centered in the chest. And if you look at senior citizens, you will often see that their breathing has moved even higher and become even shallower.

There are a number of factors at play in the progressively shallower breathing that most people experience as they age. These include:

- A major decrease in physical activity for people in our society due to modern technology and desk-based employment
- Increased stress as a result of our modern technological society (stress leads to shallower breathing)
- More time spent indoors and less engaged in outdoor activity

But perhaps the main reason is that unless you're a dancer, or an athlete, or a meditation practitioner, no one has ever taught you how to breathe. And as you get older the normal problems associated with old age make the problem worse.

☯ *Guidelines for Correct Breathing*

There are many subtleties involved in Dragon Gate breathing. However, here are a few basic guidelines that you can follow as you practice breathing correctly.

- **Relax**. The first part of the breathing process involves relaxing your body. This enables you to inhale the maximum amount of air with the minimum amount of effort. Of course, it's easy to say you should relax, and often far more difficult to accomplish, depending on what is going on in your day and in your life. This book contains a number of exercises designed to assist you in becoming more relaxed, and the process of meditation will certainly help. As your meditative breathing improves, it will carry over into your day-to-day activities.
- **Breathe in through the nose**. Ideally, you should breathe

in through the nose. The nose has a screen of hairs that traps dust, tiny insects, and other particles. The long nasal passage also is lined with mucus membranes that warm cool air and capture fine dust particles. And of course the nose provides the body's sense of smell, so breathing through the nose allows you to detect if the air you are breathing is unhealthy. (If your nose is clogged due to illness or some other issue, you will, of course, need to breathe through your mouth.)

- **Maintain good posture**. Slouching and poor posture will cut off your supply of air, just as bending a hose will cut off the supply of water. For optimal breathing, keep your back straight, chin down, and eyes level. Your shoulders should align with your hips. Keep your shoulders back and try to expand your chest cavity to give your lungs their greatest potential to expand.

- **Breathe from your abdomen**. When babies are in the womb they breathe through the umbilical cord attached to their abdomen. Once they are born they begin using their lungs, but you can still see a baby's stomach expand and contract as he or she breathes in and out. By learning to breathe from the abdomen you can fill your lungs with more air by creating space for them to expand. In the Taoist Inner Elixir school, this was often referred to as "embryonic breathing."

The best way to practice your breathing is through meditation. During meditation you will spend an extended period of time practicing the relaxed, controlled, deep breathing that will become your standard mode of breathing.

Concentrate on the goal of meditation.
Do not listen with your ear, but listen with your mind;
Not with your mind, but with your breath.
Let the hearing stop with your ear,
Let the mind stop with its images.
Breathing means to empty oneself and to wait for Tao.

—CHUANG TZU

STANDING MEDITATION

In the previous chapter you learned sitting meditation. Standing meditation can be just as relaxing as sitting meditation and can offer enhanced energy development. This is in part due to the fact that when you are standing, your body is fully elongated, unlike sitting where you are creating two significant near 90-degree angles in your hips and knees that affect energy circulation. In addition, standing provides a stronger connection to the earth. (The ideal location to stand is barefoot on the exposed ground, but of course this is only if your situation allows for this. Ultimately the best location for you is one that works for you.) Like sitting meditation, the standing meditation is extremely simple and all you need is a place to stand upright.

- Find a comfortable, flat place to stand. This can be inside or outside, but you should make sure that there are no major distractions such as noise, weather, etc.
- Make sure that you are wearing loose, comfortable clothing and that nothing is binding your abdomen.
- Stand with your feet shoulder-width apart. (You can wear

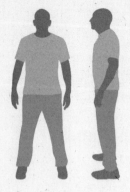

rubber-soled shoes or stand barefoot—whichever is most comfortable.) Your toes should be pointing straight ahead, or out just slightly. Your knees should be slightly bent (just not straight). Your shoulders, hips, and ankles should be aligned. Keep your back straight. Your head should be straight, eyes looking straight ahead, chin parallel to the ground.

- Try to stand as though you are sitting on the edge of a tall bar stool. In other words, you feel slightly supported even though you are not.

- Allow your arms to hang naturally by your side (but avoid allowing your shoulders to roll forward).

- Close your eyes halfway and meditate for 5 minutes. (If you feel comfortable closing your eyes while standing you may do that as well. Some people feel dizzy or lose their balance when standing up with their eyes closed.) You may set a timer but we recommend using a very soothing and quiet tone as the alarm sound. Five minutes is the beginning duration. Over time, you can extend your meditation until you are doing 10, 15, 30, or more minutes.

> Breathing out—
> Touching the root of heaven, one's heart opens.
> The dragon slips into the water.
> Breathing In—
> Standing on the root of earth, one's heart is still and deep.
> The Tiger's claw cannot be moved.
>
> —CHANG SAN-FENG

Dantian

Breathing from the abdomen holds a very special place in all Chinese meditative and martial traditions, including Taoist breathing. This is because the abdomen is the location of the point known as the dantian (tan-tien). *Dantian* literally means "cinnabar field." Cinnabar is mercury sulfide (HgS), the common ore mineral of mercury, which was traditionally viewed as an element in the Chinese (and Western) alchemy that turned lead into gold. Since the Taoist alchemy used these concepts as metaphors for a physical transformation, the cinnabar field is an essential aspect in Taoist alchemy. In Taoist internal alchemy, the dantian is also often translated as "elixir field" and is frequently referred to as the cauldron, because it is the place where the practitioner gathers, mixes, and cooks his or her sexual, vital, and spiritual energies. (You will find more on the Taoist alchemy in Chapter 7, "Dragon Gate Sexual Yoga.")

According to principles of Taoist alchemy, the body has three dantians, which function as psychic and energy centers within the body:

- The upper dantian is in the head just behind a point directly between the eyebrows and corresponds to the third eye. (In Western anatomy, this point corresponds to the pituitary gland.)
- The middle dantian is in the heart.
- The lower dantian is located at the navel (equivalent to the yogic navel chakra). For Taoist practitioners this is the most important dantian because it is the focus for the majority of

breathing exercises and meditation. In this book, when we refer to the dantian we are referring to the navel (unless specifically stated otherwise).

Many forms of Chinese martial arts as well as Buddhist and Taoist teachings hold that the dantian is located three finger widths *below* the navel—that is, about one and a half inches below the belly button. Dragon Gate, however, holds that the dantian is at the navel, three finger widths *inside* the body. Considering that this is the point from which you originally breathed as a baby in utero, this makes sense, given the Taoist emphasis on breathing like a newborn baby. It also correlates with other esoteric systems that believe in energy development, such as Indian yoga. However, given the dominance of the idea that the dantian is located below the navel, this can be a somewhat controversial opinion. My own experience has shown that conceiving the dantian as being inside, behind the navel is more natural.

The navel dantian is the main focal point for internal meditative techniques and energy development exercises for all Chinese martial arts and chi gung (chi development exercises) as well as Buddhist and Taoist meditation. A common technique in meditation is to center the mind in the dantian, which can help to physically center the practitioner as well as assist in the control of thoughts and emotions.

Dantian Meditation

The following meditation exercise will activate and energize your dantian. It takes only a couple of minutes to complete.

1. Find a comfortable, flat place to stand. This can be inside or outside, but you should make sure that there are no major distractions such as noise, weather, etc.
2. Make sure that you are wearing loose, comfortable clothing and that nothing is binding your abdomen.
3. Stand with your feet shoulder width apart. (You can wear rubber-soled shoes or sneakers or stand barefoot—whichever is most comfortable.)
4. Allow your body to relax completely.
5. Visualize the sun shining in the sky above you. Then see the sun change into a shining golden ball. Once you clearly see the golden ball in your mind's eye, swallow it and imagine it moving down your throat and into your abdomen where it settles at your dantian—a point inside the body at the level of your navel.
6. Now visualize the golden ball dividing into two. The first golden ball stays at your dantian. The second golden ball moves beside it. Now visualize the second golden ball circling around the ball at the dantian, as the planets orbit the sun. First see the second ball circle around the dantian on a horizontal plane (parallel to the ground). The second ball should circle around the dantian 3 times to the left (counterclockwise) and three times to the right (clockwise).
7. Next visualize the second golden ball circling around the dantian on a vertical plane (perpendicular to the ground). The second ball should circle around the dantian 3 times to the left (counterclockwise) and three times to the right (clockwise).
8. Take 3 deep breaths to conclude.

Chi

Chi—the energy that sustains all life—holds the key to health and longevity.

—CHRISTIANE NORTHRUP, M.D.

The dantian is of critical importance in Taoism, because it is the center of the body for the development of chi (qi) or internal energy. The concept of chi, and the breathing exercises that facilitate its development, are an essential aspect of Chinese culture.

According to traditional Chinese medicine the human body's functioning is supported by a vital energy called chi which flows through a series of channels, known as meridians, that roughly correspond to the circulatory and nervous systems. This inner force can be referred to as energy, metabolism, stamina, and it is a person's source of power, endurance, vitality, resilience, and good health. According to Taoist philosophy, chi is the essential ingredient in establishing, maintaining, and promoting good health. A strong, vigorous, healthy person has a strong chi. On a cosmic level chi is the energy behind heaven and earth that provides the impetus for perpetual change.

A baby is born with a tremendous amount of chi, which allows it to grow an ounce a day. But as human beings age, the amount of energy within the body begins to decline. To the Chinese, the condition of a person's chi determines the physical condition of the body. A strong, vigorous, healthy person has a strong chi. The purpose of Taoist breathing exercises is to strengthen the chi.

Chi is also the essential ingredient in Taoist spiritual development. The development of the chi within the body represents an attempt to fully balance and integrate the microcosmic universe within man with the macrocosmic universe outside.

Consequently, it is the force that enables you to follow the Taoist alchemical path. Additionally, by becoming sensitive to the flow of chi within yourself, you become sensitive to the chi in the world around you, which provides insight into the nature of reality.

It is important to note that chi is not a mysterious force that affects the body, like the ether of the medieval alchemists. Traditional Chinese medicine is based on the idea that we have natural patterns of chi that circulate throughout our bodies. Illness is believed to be the product of disrupted, blocked, unbalanced, or insufficient chi. Traditional Chinese medicine attempts to cure illness by adjusting the circulation of chi using methods that include herbal medicines, special diets, moxibustion (a technique that involves the burning of mugwort on an acupuncture point to facilitate healing), massage, and acupuncture. However, to generate more chi, the traditional prescription has always been to practice chi development exercises, or chi gung (qi gong), such as the ones presented in this book. There are also exercises that are used to treat specific maladies.

Taoist breathing exercises are specifically designed to cultivate the chi. *The Yellow Emperor's Classic of Internal Medicine* contains a chapter called "Natural Truth in Ancient Times" that says:

When one is completely free of wishes or ambition, he will really get the genuine vital energy. When one concentrates his consciousness internally, how can diseases attack him? One must breathe the essence of life, defend oneself independently by regulating one's respiration to preserve one's spirit and make the muscles remain unchanged.

Taoist breathing exercises involve the combination of both inner and outer strengthening. This union of internal and external is regarded as essential to bring yin and yang into harmony. In essence the concept of the Tao suggests a return to a fundamental union of Heaven, Earth, and Man. The passive and active principles of yin and yang are not antagonistic but mutually complementary parts of a greater whole. Health and longevity stem from a balanced and harmonious interaction of yin and yang. The sage who could maintain the balance by flowing with the cyclical currents of perpetual change was assured of a long life and attainment of Tao.

> If one desires to cultivate the path of immortals, one must first cultivate the path of men. As long as the path of men has not yet been cultivated, the path of immortals will be far. The Confucians say that only after having harmonized one's family can one pacify the country. Harmonizing the family corresponds to the path of men, and pacifying the country to the path of immortals.
>
> —WANG KUNYANG

Taoists sought immortality by cultivating their chi. According to traditional Taoist literature, the dantian is the reservoir of the chi in the body and when it overflows the chi permeates the bones and aging ceases as the energy of the universe and the energy of man become one. As the vital principle of the nervous system, chi circulates through the body in regular cycles. It is the perpetual current of energy that flows between yin and yang. When chi is properly channeled and concentrated it can become an enormous source of strength.

Developing a Free Flow of Chi

What follows is a series of Dragon Gate breathing exercises specifically designed to promote Taoist breathing and stimulate the development of chi. Initially, the changes that occur when practicing in this manner are subtle, requiring practice over an extended period of time (which varies according to the individual). The key is not how long the individual trains, but how regularly.

The following two exercises are essential Dragon Gate practices designed to quickly stimulate a free flow of chi within your body. They are very powerful.

FULL-BODY BREATHING

1. You may do this exercise either standing or sitting (though standing is preferable). First follow the instructions (previously given) for standing or sitting meditation, depending on which method you prefer.
2. Allow your body to relax completely.
3. Inhale, slowly and deeply, and as you do imagine that your entire body is breathing in. That is, air is being breathed in from every part of your body.
4. Exhale slowly and deeply, and as you do, imagine that your entire body is breathing out. That is, air is being breathed out from every part of your body.
5. Do this for 5 minutes. (You may extend the time if you feel comfortable with the practice.)
6. The key to this exercise is clearly imagining your entire body

engaged in the breathing process. If you have any difficulty in imagining your entire body engaged in breathing (as opposed to just your lungs), just do your best. Over time, it will become easier.

Creating Your Energy Ball

1. You may do this exercise either standing or sitting (though standing is preferable). First follow the instructions for standing or sitting meditation, depending on which method you prefer.
2. Allow your body to relax completely.
3. Inhale and exhale slowly and deeply and as you breathe feel the energy you are gathering at your dantian spreading around your body like a force field.
4. As the exercise progresses, feel yourself existing in a void, floating in space in a ball of energy.
5. Do this for 5 minutes. (You may extend the time if you feel comfortable with the practice.)
6. To close, feel the energy ball gather together and fold into your dantian.
7. The key to this exercise is clearly imagining your entire body in a ball of energy. If you have any difficulty in imagining yourself in an energy ball, just do your best. Over time, it will become easier.

Accessing Chi from Nature

I urge you to bring into harmony for me nature, heaven, and Tao. There must be an end and a beginning. Heaven must be in accord with the lights of the sky, the celestial bodies and their course and periods. The earth below must reflect the four seasons, the five elements, that which is precious and that which is lowly and without value—one as well as the other. Is it not that in winter man responds to yin (the principle of darkness and cold)? And is it not that in summer he responds to yang (the principle of light and warmth)?

—*The Yellow Emperor's Classic of Internal Medicine*

As noted earlier, Taoism is based on the idea that humanity is a microcosm of the universe and so we may gain knowledge of the universe by going within. The opposite is also true. Since we are a microcosm of the natural world, we can gain knowledge, energy, and power from the world around us. In this way, we can draw chi from nature.

Taoism has always emphasized a return to nature's harmony as a means of self-transcendence. Dragon Gate seeks union with the Tao by physical and mental emulation of the forces of nature such as yin and yang and the five elements and though the exercises shown in this book can be practiced anywhere, special benefits can be had by drawing energy from the forces of heaven (the sky, including the sun, moon, clouds, and wind) and earth (including everything on the earth such as trees, plants, bodies of water, and rocks).

The natural location you select is important. So, find a place that suits you, one that seems to be your special spot. Focus on elements of nature that attract you the most as well as ones that are easily accessible. Remember that when you are outside, you should be as comfortable as possible in order to enhance relaxation and to enter a deeper state of meditation. Therefore, choose a comfortable, flat space (especially if you are doing standing meditation), and make sure that you are neither too cold nor too hot. Early morning and late afternoon are typically very powerful times to do these nature practices, but you may find it useful to practice at midday or at night depending on how the energy feels for you.

You may do these exercises at any time of year (assuming you can make yourself comfortable). You can attune yourself to the different energies that are available at the different seasons.

If suitable conditions are not readily available, these exercises can be performed from inside your home, so long as you have a good view of (and, if possible, can hear) that natural power which you are tapping into.

Once you have become comfortable with working with any of the forces of nature, you can tap into that same power at any time by simply re-creating the thoughts, feelings, and physical state that you experience during the meditation while you are elsewhere. In this way, you can use natural forces to assist with your practice at any time and place.

> When you become one with nature, you are in accord with the Tao.
>
> —LAO TZU

What follows are two Dragon Gate exercises designed to enable you to quickly integrate the power of nature into your practice. Each natural force has its own characteristics. For instance, the sun is powerful, trees are deeply rooted and live a very long time, the oceans move mountains over time, and so on. You can work with these obvious characteristics as well as going deeper and seeking out the special essence within each element. In selecting the natural force you wish to use in your practice you may open yourself to a variety of objects in an area and allow your personal power to direct you to the specific one that is best for you to work with at that moment in time.

UNITING WITH THE FORCES OF HEAVEN

1. You may do this exercise standing, sitting, or lying down (though standing is generally preferable for energy development). The key here is to make yourself completely comfortable. Make sure that the ground you are on is level and that you can stay comfortably in the position you have selected for a minimum of 5 minutes. Ensure that your clothing is not constricting your body and that you are not cold or uncomfortably warm.

2. Ensuring that your body is in alignment, allow yourself to relax completely.

3. For this exercise you may unite with any natural force that you perceive as being part of the heavens, including the sun (do not look directly at the sun), moon, stars, wind, clouds, rainbows, and the sky itself. If you try one and it doesn't work well for you, try it again another time. If you are still not feeling an affinity for it, try something else.

4. Spend a few moments thinking about the natural force that you have selected. Contemplate its essence and energy. Then think about it as a living, vibrant aspect of your own consciousness.

5. Feel yourself absorbing the power of the natural object you have selected. In this process use all of your senses (visual, auditory, sensual, olfactory, and gustatory) to completely capture the essence of the natural force.

6. At any point you may extend your hands, palms open, to assist in drawing in the energy. When you do this, feel a vortex of energy in the center of your palms that easily interacts with the energy around you.

7. Now merge your energy with the energy that you perceive as being intrinsic to the natural force you are working with. For something like the sun, this power is obvious, but by exploring the natural powers you will find that they each have their own unique essence and energy that you can tap into.

8. Spend 5 minutes in this practice (you may extend the time as you wish).

9. To conclude, if you have extended your hands, close the energy vortex in your palms and bring your arms to your sides. Then bring the energy you have gathered to your dantian and take 3 very deep breaths.

The key to this exercise is opening yourself to the natural force that you are using.

UNITING WITH THE FORCES OF THE EARTH

1. You may do this exercise standing, sitting, or lying down (though standing is generally preferable for energy development). The key here is to make yourself completely comfort-

able. Make sure that the ground you are on is level and that you can stay comfortably in the position you have selected for a minimum of 5 minutes. Ensure that your clothing is not constricting your body and that you are not cold or uncomfortably warm.

2. Ensuring that your body is in alignment, allow yourself to relax completely.

3. For this exercise you may unite with any natural force that you perceive as being part of the earth, including the ground, trees, plants, any body of water (including lakes, rivers, oceans), rocks, and so on. (Do not use animals since they are likely to move.) If you try one and it doesn't work well for you, try it again another time. If you are still not feeling an affinity for it, try something else.

4. Spend a few moments thinking about the natural force that you have selected. Contemplate its essence and energy. Then think about it as a living, vibrant aspect of your own consciousness.

5. Feel yourself absorbing the power of the natural object you have selected. In this process use all of your senses (visual, auditory, sensual, olfactory, and gustatory) to completely capture the essence of the natural force.

6. At any point you may extend your hands, palms open, to assist in drawing in the energy. When you do this, feel a vortex of energy in the center of your palms that easily interacts with the energy around you.

7. Now merge your energy with the energy that you perceive as being intrinsic to the natural force you are working with. For something like the ocean, this power is obvious, but by exploring the natural powers you will find that they

each have their own unique essence and energy that you can tap into.

8. Spend 5 minutes in this practice (you may extend the time as you wish).

9. To conclude, if you have extended your hands, close the energy vortex in your palms and bring your arms to your sides. Then bring the energy you have gathered to your dantian and take 3 very deep breaths.

The key to this exercise is opening yourself to the natural force that you are using.

In conclusion, it is important to note that while this chapter has focused on using breathwork and nature practices to develop your chi, according to Taoism, your chi can be developed and enhanced using every aspect of your life including diet, exercise, mental activities, sex, and dreaming. So while breathing is at the core of Dragon Gate chi development, keep in mind that every facet of your life affects your generation and use of chi. This book provides information on many of these methods.

Fourth Gate:
Cultivating the Mind

DRAGON GATE MEDITATION PRACTICES

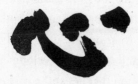

Mind

To remain hidden or to fly and leap, it is all up to the mind.

—CHANG PO-TUAN, *Understanding Reality*,
ELEVENTH CENTURY A.D.

Please take a moment now before you begin this chapter to practice this brief and simple exercise. It will help you to maximize your enjoyment of the chapter.

Lie down, relax, and close your eyes. Now become aware of the internal dialogue in your mind. Simply observe the dialogue without judgment or making any effort to direct the flow of thoughts. Do this for 1 to 2 minutes.

Now you are ready to begin.

The Power of Your Mind

Flow with whatever may happen and let your mind be free. Stay
centered by accepting whatever you are doing. This is the ultimate.

—CHUANG TZU

In the previous chapter we looked at the importance of breathing
and meditation to develop your chi. But the development of chi is
not an end in itself. Once you have learned how to breathe correctly,
the next step is to use those breathing methods in conjunction with
meditation practices to stimulate greater chi flow with the goal
being rapid mental and spiritual development. This is part of a
process of self-cultivation that lies at the core of Dragon Gate practice and philosophy. The ultimate goal of the practice is the libera-
tion of the mind and the development of intuitive consciousness.

Taoists believe that the physical reality we perceive is a projection
of our consciousness. As noted in the Yi Jing (I Ching), the essential manual on the functioning of the universe: "The auspicious
and the ominous, both arise from the same circumstances." Essentially, this is stating that how we choose to perceive "reality" creates
the experience of reality that we have—or that there is no objective
reality.

The idea that our perception of reality is of primary importance
is captured by a famous Zen story:

Two traveling monks, a teacher and his student, reached a rapidly
flowing river, where they met a young woman. Wary of the current,
she asked if they could help her across.

"We are sorry, kind lady," said the student. "A monk is not
allowed to touch a woman." But the teacher, having compassion for

her, offered to carry her on his back and, lifting her, proceeded to wade across the water. He put her down on the opposite bank. She thanked him, and the two monks went on their way.

The monks continued on in silence. But the younger monk was upset by his teacher's actions. Finally, unable to hold his silence, he turned to his teacher and said, "Master, you know we have taken vows and are not supposed to touch women. How could you carry that woman like that?"

"My dear student," the master replied, "I did carry that woman across the river. But there I put her down while you are apparently still carrying her."

There is a simple but powerful metaphor that you can use in attempting to think about this concept, which is to view your life as a play in which you are the actor as well as the author of the play. The "you" that is the actor functions as an independent being, typically unaware of how the world you exist in is a creation of your consciousness. You are also unaware of your author self. The author self creates this play for the actor self to experience. The experiences are created without judgment, so while you may assign great value to certain aspects of your reality, the author self has created it all and so does not view any portion of the reality as being inherently superior to any other. Of course, the author self certainly recognizes that the actor self will perceive certain elements of reality as being more desirable than others.

People can often easily comprehend how they have created the good things in their lives, but they can have far more difficulty in seeing how they have created those elements of their lives that they are not happy with—those that cause pain and suffering. In other words, they don't perceive themselves as creating their own reality.

This is completely understandable, but, from the Taoist perspective, is the result of faulty thinking, and the result of viewing their reality with judgment rather than as an experience.

Ultimately, any experience is perceived to be good or bad based only on the judgment we assign to it. We can view a movie filled with violence and find it thrilling and entertaining. But if we were told that the same movie was a documentary film about violence that had actually occurred, we might very well be horrified. Now you may say, but one is fiction and one is fact and so they are very different, and you would be right. But life is filled with experiences that seemed bad at the time, but ultimately led to something wonderful occurring. For instance, you lose your job and you perceive your career to be over when suddenly a new door opens. And the opposite is also true. Something that can seem wonderful can quickly turn into a nightmare. This is why Lao Tzu says: "Be careful what you water your dreams with. Water them with worry and fear and you will produce weeds that choke the life from your dream. Water them with optimism and solutions and you will cultivate success. Always be on the lookout for ways to turn a problem into an opportunity for success. Always be on the lookout for ways to nurture your dream."

In seeking to understand this concept it is again useful to turn to a famous Zen story called "Maybe":

Once there was an old farmer whose horse ran away. Upon hearing the news, his neighbors came to visit. "Such bad luck," they said sympathetically.

"Maybe," the farmer said.

The next morning the horse returned, bringing with it three other wild horses. "How wonderful," the neighbors exclaimed.

"Maybe," the farmer said.

The following day, his son tried to ride one of the untamed horses, was thrown, and broke his leg. The neighbors again came to offer their sympathy on his misfortune.

"Maybe," the farmer said.

The day after, military officials came to the village to draft young men into the army. Seeing that the son's leg was broken, they passed him by. The neighbors congratulated the farmer on how well things had turned out.

"Maybe," the farmer said.

From the Taoist perspective, which sees the physical universe as the infinite interplay of yin and yang, there can be no happiness without the existence of unhappiness since each element of reality is defined by its opposite. It is only once we have completely unified with the Tao, or all that is, that we are freed from this basic law of the universe and we move from dualistic consciousness (yin/yang, self/other) to unitary consciousness where everything is perceived as being Tao.

It is important to note that the belief in one's authorship of one's own reality is specifically intended to help free you from fears and empower you to deal with your reality. It is *not* meant to be a vehicle to self-destructive tendencies. So it is very important that you:

1. Don't victimize yourself because you are not happy with the reality you have created. Knowledge of your creatorhood is meant to enhance your appreciation of your reality. Even when things appear to go "badly," it's important to remember the awesome power involved in the creation of reality and how it flows in keeping with the Tao. Avoid beating

yourself up because things aren't going your way. As Lao Tzu wrote: "Failure is an opportunity."

2. Don't become egotistical and believe that the world around you and everyone in it is a figment of your mind and therefore you can treat it and them however you wish because they have no objective existence of their own. This reality is yours to experience and to cherish. The people who appear in your reality are meant to be treated with compassion.

3. Don't frighten yourself. If you believe that your thoughts create your reality, it is possible to become frightened of your creative abilities. What if you think something bad about a person or yourself? Thoughts are not dangerous. However, if you focus on those thoughts, nurture them, and give them weight, then you may take the actions necessary to bring those thoughts into reality. So don't be afraid of your thoughts, good, bad, or neutral. They are your creations. Enjoy them and have fun with them.

Admittedly, the idea of conscious creatorhood can be somewhat controversial and challenging. It is only natural to question a concept that implies that people have created the "bad" things that have occurred to them—including horrible, nightmarish tragedies. Clearly, people do not actively and consciously want bad things to happen to them, and yet bad things still do happen.

Ultimately, this concept is not one that can be proven. But the idea is part of Taoist and most other spiritual traditions. However, all the essential benefits to be had from the Taoist practices described in this book do not require a belief in conscious creatorhood. If the concept works for you, then use it. If it doesn't, then feel free to ignore it. Whatever your view, it is always good practice to question any concept. Indeed the process of questioning is an excellent mental practice in and of itself.

PRELIMINARY MENTAL PRACTICES

> Such moments when Mind and Matter hold perfect communion
> And wide vistas open to regions hitherto entirely barred,
> Will come with irresistible force,
> And go, their departure none can hinder.
> Hiding, they vanish like a flash of light;
> Manifest, they are like sounds arising in midair.
>
> —LU CHI, CHINESE SCHOLAR, A.D. 261–303

In order to create the reality you desire and to find a path that makes for a rewarding journey, you need to cultivate your mental powers. This is accomplished through meditation practices designed to strengthen, focus, and develop your mind.

Dragon Gate has created an advanced system for the expansion of your mind's inherent abilities that combines breathing exercises, visualizations, and advanced thought experiments. In the previous chapter you learned the basic meditation exercises that are at the core of mental development. In this chapter you will learn additional visualization and thought exercises that when combined with the chi development and calming exercises create a powerful platform for mental development.

Note: If you have any difficulty in doing any of the mental exercises outlined in this chapter, don't worry about it. The purpose of these exercises is to enhance your experience of reality, not to cause frustration. If practicing an exercise gets too frustrating, you can try to simply imagine that you are doing the exercise easily. And if that doesn't work, skip the exercise and move on. Just do the best that you can. With practice it will get much easier.

DRAGON GATE INTRODUCTORY VISUALIZATION PRACTICE

Choose a small object that you are familiar with. This should be something that you can hold in your hands, preferably an article that you see and/or use every day. (A vase, an article of clothing, a pen, a watch, etc.)

1. Find a comfortable place to sit. This can be inside or outside, but you should make sure that there are no major distractions such as noise, weather, etc. There should be a table or flat surface in front of you on which you can place your article so that you can easily observe it with your head level (not looking up or down).
2. Place the article on the table in front of you.
3. Close your eyes and take 3 deep breaths.
4. Now open your eyes and completely take in the object for 1 or 2 minutes. You should attempt to see every facet of the object (length, width, color, size, shape, texture). But while doing this it is important that you continue breathing deeply and stay completely relaxed. So observe the object, but do your best not to study it in a manner that would cause tension or stress.
5. Now close your eyes and visualize the object for 1 to 2 minutes. Attempt to re-create in your mind's eye the same object in all its facets and dimensions.

6. Use this same object on subsequent practice sessions until you are completely comfortable with it and then do the exercise without the object in front of you.

DRAGON GATE THOUGHT EXPERIMENT: ENCOUNTER WITH THE AUTHOR SELF

1. Find a comfortable place to sit or lie down. This can be inside or outside, but you should make sure that there are no major distractions such as noise, weather, etc.
2. Close your eyes and take 3 deep breaths.
3. Think about any event in your life. It can be something that happened to you recently, or something from your past. The only requirement is that you have a good, vivid recall of the event.
4. Re-create the event in your mind from the perspective of the actor self. That is, identify yourself completely with the character in the world you visualize who is you. Activate as many senses in this experience as you can (sight, sound, taste, smell, touch). Spend a couple of minutes in this state.
5. Now re-create the exact same event in your mind from the perspective of the author self. That is, identify yourself as the author of the experience including the complete power to have chosen the location, all the characters who appear, and all the actions that take place. Spend a couple of minutes in this state.

The Power of Meditation

The scholar learns something every day. The man of Tao unlearns
something every day, until he gets back to non-doing.

—LAO TZU

The regular practice of meditation provides numerous benefits,
which include improved mental clarity, sharper memory, reduced
stress, better sleep cycles, and greater enjoyment of life. But while
these subjective measures can be experienced by anyone who
chooses to practice meditation for even just a few weeks, elements
of the scientific community have been attempting to measure the
benefits of meditation in a systematic way. While the transformed
states brought about by meditation have traditionally been understood in transcendent terms, as something outside the world of
physical measurement and objective evaluation, scientists have
found a variety of fascinating methods to analyze and quantify the
experience.

These Western "scientific" studies of meditation and other types
of contemplative practice began in the 1930s when Kovoor Behanan, an Indian graduate student in psychology at Yale University,
undertook the first empirical study of yoga and meditation. With
the help of his teacher, Dr. Walter Miles, Behanan began a basic
analysis of oxygen consumption during meditation and yogic
breathing exercises. His work, which found an increase in oxygen
consumption, helped stimulate additional experiments.

In the 1970s, with the popularization of the Maharishi's tran-
scendental meditation technique (owing to the Beatles' promotion
of it) as well as the advent of the "new age" movement, the scientific
study of meditation really took off. But soon meditation studies lost

a lot of their popularity until there was a resurgence of interest in mind-body science in the mid-1990s.

The new popularity of brain research has been spurred on in part by a growing awareness of the role mental states—and stress in particular—play in health and recovery. But the increase in popularity is also the result of major advances in technology, such as brain imaging, that have made it possible to see what is happening inside the brain and explore the biology of mental processes. That's why the majority of breakthroughs in brain sciences have happened in the last fifteen years—including the discovery that brain cells are constantly created and connecting to each other, even late in life. The effects of meditation on psychological factors, such as depression and anxiety, have also been measured using sophisticated psychological testing techniques. There are a large number of studies, conducted by independent scientists at major universities around the world, that have discovered amazing things.

> Longtime [meditation] practitioners showed brain activation on a scale we have never seen before.
>
> —RICHARD DAVIDSON, PH.D.

For instance, numerous studies have shown that meditators use a larger percentage of their brains. Of particular note is the groundbreaking work by Dr. Richard Davidson, professor of psychiatry and psychology at the University of Wisconsin's Keck Laboratory for Functional Brain Imaging and Behavior. Using advanced brain imaging technology, he and others have translated the subjective mental experiences of meditation into objective waveforms. According to Dr. Davidson, meditators' "mental practice is having an effect on the brain in the same way golf or tennis practice will enhance performance . . . What we found is that the longtime [meditation] practitioners showed brain activation on a scale we have never seen before." His work demonstrates that the brain is capable of being trained and physically modified in ways Western medicine and science has only begun to imagine.

Other studies show that meditators actually increase the physical size of their brains. Dr. Sara Lazar at Massachusetts General Hospital has used MRI to analyze the brains of meditators and has found that "You are exercising [the brain] while you meditate, and it gets bigger." The growth of the cortex is due to wider blood vessels, more supporting structures such as glia and astrocytes, and increased branching and connections (glia and astrocytes are non-neuronal cells that provide support and protective functions in the brain). Dr. Lazar's findings match those of other studies such as one carried out at Harvard Medical School that found that brain regions involved in focusing attention and processing sense information were thicker in meditators than non-meditators. While these findings may seem astounding, they are in line with studies showing that accomplished musicians, athletes, and linguists all display growth in relevant areas of the cortex. Albert Einstein's brain, for instance, showed a significantly greater quantity of glia in an area known to play an important role in abstract imagery.

Other benefits of meditation for our mental processes include improved focus, better memory function, and better cognitive abilities overall including problem solving, concentration and attention, improved reaction time, better scores on intelligence tests, greater creativity, and improved sleep.

In addition to harnessing the power of your mind, studies show that meditation carries a host of health benefits including: reduced hypertension; lower blood pressure; reduced stress, anxiety, and depression; fewer hospitalizations; enhanced immune system function; and even reduced mortality rates.

It is important to note that brain studies of meditation have a fundamental weakness shared by human research in many other fields, which is that it is impossible to rule out the effects of other variables, such as differences in language, culture, and lifestyle between meditators and control groups. It may very well be possible that long-term meditators are intrinsically different types of people. Yet the wide range of experiments and the overwhelmingly positive results, as well as the studies on people who have never meditated previously, all clearly indicate that meditation offers significant benefits. The Taoist view is that one should gain personal knowledge of this by practicing and experiencing the benefits for oneself.

DRAGON GATE THOUGHT EXPERIMENT: THE ORIGIN OF THOUGHTS

1. Find a comfortable place to sit or lie down. This can be inside or outside, but you should make sure that there are no major distractions such as noise, weather, etc.
2. Close your eyes and take 3 deep breaths.
3. Become aware of your thoughts. Allow them to arise freely, without any judgment or any attempt to stop or direct them in any way. A benefit of this particular exercise is that it can

be undertaken at any time—even when you are feeling very stressed out or excited, for there is no need to calm your mind.

4. As your thoughts flow, seek the point in your mind where the thoughts originate. Where do thoughts come from? This should be an easy process, like counting cars on the highway. There should be nothing stressful about it. If you are having any problems, try imagining that you can sense the point of origin for your thoughts. People can experience the origin of their thoughts in various ways—as images, feelings, sounds, or sensations. In some cases, you may experience the origin of a thought as something completely unexpected or unrelated to the thought itself. Whatever you experience and however you experience it, simply allow it to flow naturally.

5. Seek only the origin of your thoughts. Once you have experienced the origin of a thought, let it go and move on to the next thought. If you have a period where there are no thoughts, enjoy the profundity of the experience.

6. Do this for 3 to 5 minutes.

DRAGON GATE THOUGHT EXPERIMENT: THE TERMINATION OF THOUGHTS

This exercise is identical to the previous exercise (the origin of thoughts) except this time you will attempt to experience the termination of thoughts. As your thoughts flow, seek the point in your mind where the thoughts terminate or disappear. Where do thoughts go? Remember, if you are having any problems with this exercise, try imagining that you can sense the point of termination for your thoughts.

MEDITATION AND STRESS REDUCTION

Optimal cognitive function requires a relaxed mental state.

—DHARMA SINGH KHALSA, M.D.

It is widely agreed that meditation offers opportunities for promoting both mental and physical health. But perhaps the single most powerful reason to meditate is its proven ability to reduce stress and anxiety.

The modern world we live in offers many technological toys and physical comforts. However, it has also created an environment with an amazing amount of stress brought on by everything from pollution, environmental toxins, noise, and information overload to the relentless struggle to survive and succeed.

A mild degree of stress can be beneficial for the brain. It causes the release of norepinephrine, a neurotransmitter that creates a positive mood and also moves short-term memory to long-term storage. It also helps the brain grow new dendrites (dendrites, from the Greek word for tree, are the branched filaments in neurons that conduct the electrochemical signals from other neurons) and create new synaptic pathways (associated with improved memory and mental function). However, when you endure stress on a regular basis, your body generates excess cortisol. Cortisol, also known as the stress hormone, is secreted by the adrenal glands. Its primary function is to increase blood sugar and stores of sugar in the liver. But it is also involved in regulating numerous other bodily functions including blood pressure, insulin release for blood sugar maintenance, immune function, and inflammatory response.

Normally, cortisol is present in the body at higher levels in the morning, and it is at its lowest at night. It's also secreted in higher levels during the body's fight-or-flight response to stress. The release of cortisol has some positive effects, such as providing a quick burst of energy, enhancing mental functions such as memory and thought processing, and reducing sensitivity to pain.

Unfortunately, prolonged periods with elevated levels of cortisol has been documented to cause numerous significant health problems including high blood pressure, blood sugar imbalances, reduced immune function, and impaired mental performance. Studies have also shown that people who secrete higher levels of cortisol in response to stress also tend to eat more food (and less healthy food) than people who secrete less cortisol. Consequently, the result of excess cortisol can be heart attacks, strokes, obesity, and a variety of other physical and mental illnesses.

Perhaps most significantly, excess cortisol has been shown to actually kill neurons (neurons are cells in the nervous system that process and transmit information). In other words, it destroys your brain. This can be experienced as memory loss, an inability to think clearly, making rash decisions, premature senility, etc. That's why people under heavy stress find it hard to concentrate and think clearly. Unfortunately, as stress causes cognitive problems, people tend to compensate by pushing themselves even harder, resulting in a degenerative cycle.

Studies show that even very intelligent people become markedly less rational as their stress levels increase. More recently the direct relationship between stress and elevated cortisol levels has been clearly demonstrated. Numerous studies, including those of Dr. Herbert Benson of Harvard University (often referred to as the father of mind-body medicine) and Dr. Robert Sapolsky of Stanford University have revealed a strong correlation between high levels of cortisol (caused by stress) and mental decline.

A key finding of this research is that keeping cortisol levels low apparently preserves brain health and cognitive skills. So the mental decline that we may have been programmed to expect as we get older is not an inevitable part of aging, but is largely due to chronic cortisol overload. If you lower your stress, you will lower your cortisol levels and your brain will regenerate its powers to learn and remember. Several studies of senior citizens have shown that those who have low cortisol levels perform as well as younger people on cognitive tests.

So what can you do to reduce stress and cortisol secretion? The main recommendations of health authorities using both Western and Eastern modalities is to follow the guidelines on living a healthy life, laid out in Chapter 2. These include proper diet and physical exercise. But a central aspect of the process is learning how to relax your mind and one of the best ways to do this is through meditation. Studies have clearly shown that during meditation blood pressure and muscle tension decrease, brain waves slow, immune system function is enhanced, blood flow to the brain increases, and alertness and memory are improved. Perhaps most importantly, during meditation, cortisol levels in the body decrease. It has also been documented that regular meditation does have an antiaging effect.

Perhaps the best way to sum it up is using Dr. Benson's phrase that the fully relaxed mind is the "magical mind."

Food for Thought

Nourish yourself internally.
In peace, stillness and complete emptiness,
The hidden light of the origin will glow
To illuminate the entire body.

—WEI PO YANG, *The Triplex Unity*
(A CLASSIC SECOND-CENTURY ALCHEMICAL TEXT)

As mentioned, the key elements for keeping your brain healthy and your mental functioning at optimum levels are the health keys outlined in Chapter 2. Essentially, brain health programs are the same as body health programs. So, proper breathing, hydration, nutrition, exercise, sleep, and meditation all have the potential to improve our brain health and mental functioning. Consequently, if you are having any kinds of problems with your mental functions (memory, thinking clearly, irritability, anxiety, etc.) you can know that making changes in these areas is a viable strategy for enhancing cognitive abilities, protecting the brain from damage, and counteracting the effects of aging. There are of course many other factors and there are foods and exercises specifically designed to improve your mental health.

First, let's take a look at some basic facts about the brain, which is the most complex organ in your body.

- Structure. The brain is made of three main parts: the forebrain, midbrain, and hindbrain. The forebrain consists of the cerebrum, thalamus, and hypothalamus. The midbrain consists of the tectum and tegmentum. The hindbrain is made of the cerebellum, pons, and medulla.

- Size. Average dimensions of the adult brain: width 5.5 in., length 6.5 in., height 3.6 in.
- Weight. At birth our brains weigh an average of 4–5 lbs., as adults the brain averages about 3 lbs. After age thirty, the brain shrinks 0.25 percent in mass each year.
- Composition. The brain is composed of 77 to 78 percent water, 10 to 12 percent fat, 8 percent protein, 1 percent carbohydrates, 2 percent soluble organics, and 1 percent inorganic salt.
- Your brain is about 2 percent of your total body weight but uses 20 percent of your body's energy.
- There are about 100 billion neurons in the human brain, the same number of stars in our galaxy.
- The left hemisphere of the brain has 186 million more neurons than the right hemisphere.
- Ten seconds is the amount of time until unconsciousness after the loss of blood supply to the brain. The brain can stay alive for 4 to 6 minutes without oxygen, after which cells begin to die.
- More electrical impulses are generated in one day by a single human brain than by all the telephones in the world.

☯ Nutrition

Food is like a pharmaceutical compound that affects the brain.

—Dr. Fernando Gómez-Pinilla, Ph.D.,
Division of Neurosurgery and
Department of Physiological Science

One of the keys of brain health and one of the things that is easiest to change is nutrition. If you're noticing any of your mental abilities slowing down, the first place to look is your diet. You need to keep your brain fueled with the proper energy and provide it with plenty of raw material to build and repair itself.

☯ *Antioxidants*

Antioxidants have probably received the most attention of all the nutritional elements that are being investigated for fighting mental decline. These include vitamins A, C, E, and polyphenols (which are found in many fruits, vegetables, whole grains, and other foods such as red wine, coffee, and chocolate), all of which reduce oxidative damage to cells. In its simplest terms, oxidation can be thought of as the biological equivalent of rusting. It's a chemical process in which two or more substances interact resulting in the loss of at least one electron. The effect is that you have atoms and molecules with unpaired electrons that are highly chemically reactive. These "free radicals" as they are called, are believed to cause cell damage (including injury to our DNA) and have been associated with a wide variety of illnesses and health problems such as cancer, heart disease, atherosclerosis, and Parkinson's disease. Some scientists believe that free radicals are the fundamental cause of aging itself.

Antioxidants can be found in large quantities in most berries (typically the blue/purple/red fruits such as acai and blueberry have the most), most other fruits, most vegetables (especially the dark green ones), whole grains, nuts, and seeds. For those of you who want to have a little extra fun with your antioxidants, they can also be found in red wine, coffee, chocolate (the darker the better), tea (especially green tea), and honey.

☯ *Omega-3 Fatty Acids*

After antioxidants, omega-3 fatty acids (EPA, DHA, and ALA) have emerged as the dietary compound that appears to be most helpful in enhancing learning and memory and preventing mental disorders. Omega-3 oils work directly on the brain, nourishing cell membranes and increasing the strength of connections between brain cells.

Dr. Fernando Gómez-Pinilla of the the Neurotrophic Research Laboratory at the UCLA Division of Neurosurgery and Department of Physiological Science has been studying the effects of food on the brain for years. According to Dr. Gómez-Pinilla, "Omega-3 fatty acids are essential for normal brain function. Dietary deficiency of omega-3 fatty acids in humans has been associated with increased risk of several mental disorders, including attention-deficit disorder, dyslexia, dementia, depression, bipolar disorder, and schizophrenia."

Your body cannot make omega-3 oils from other compounds, so it's important for you to eat foods rich in them. These oils are found in fish and certain seeds and nuts. The best sources of omega-3s are mackerel, herring, sardines, salmon, anchovies, whitefish, and sablefish. Whenever possible, eat wild-caught fish, as opposed to farm raised. Farm-raised fish are much fattier, provide less usable beneficial omega-3 fatty acids, and are typically exposed to antibiotics, pesticides, and carcinogenic chemicals such as PCBs.

The major difference between omega-3s derived from fish oils versus vegetarian sources is that the vegetarian source (such as flax seed oil) provides only ALA, but not DHA or EPA. (ALA, or alpha-linolenic acid, is short-chain omega-3 found in plant sources. It is believed that the body needs to convert the short-chain version to a long-chain version in order to make complete use of it. EPA, or eicosapentaenoic acid, and DHA, or docosahexaenoic acid, are considered long-chain omega-3s and are found in fish and algae.) So fish oil (either from wild-caught fish, or supplements derived from wild-caught fish) is the best way to get all your omega-3s. But if you're a vegetarian, getting omega-3s from a vegetarian source is certainly better than none at all.

🜨 *Additional Nutritional Factors*

- Limit your sugar (and more importantly your high fructose corn syrup) intake. Controlling levels of glucose in the blood is believed to help protect memory and cognitive function.
- Limit your alcohol intake. Studies have shown that while low to moderate levels of alcohol consumption helps protect you from cardiovascular disease, heavy drinking shrinks brains.
- Limit your intake of toxins, whether they are environmental or food- and drug-based. Toxic substances cause a host of problems, from cancer to brain damage. (This is why when it comes to choosing your food, it's always best to opt for organic produce and free-range meat that do not have pesticides, preservatives, and hormones that can offset the food's benefits.)
- Reduce the amount of food you eat. Numerous studies have shown the benefits of calorie reduction in promoting overall health and longevity as well as cognitive functions.

Exercising Your Mind

Whenever you read a book or have a conversation, the experience causes physical changes in your brain.

—GEORGE JOHNSON, *In the Palaces of Memory*

Studies have shown that it is possible to exercise your cognitive functions such as memory, sensory perception, cognition, and decision making just as you exercise your body. In fact, mental activity actually causes physical changes in your brain just as lifting weights causes your muscles to grow. The more we use our brains, the better our brains function and the bigger they become.

Exercising your brain offers many benefits and can increase your memory, protect you from dementia, and sharpen concentration. In considering a program of brain training, many of the same considerations as a physical exercise program apply. These include:

- The exercises must be challenging. You will need to continually increase the level of challenge in your exercises if you want to grow.
- The exercises must be varied. Once you have become too familiar with an exercise, it will lose some of its effectiveness. Then it's time to move on. That's why it's a good idea to keep trying new things all throughout your life. Some things to try are taking a class, studying a new instrument, and seeking out new social groups to participate in.
- Use different exercises to focus on separate cognitive abilities. Whatever the mental faculty, there are exercises specifically designed to strengthen it.

☯ Pay Attention

Perhaps the single best and easiest thing you can learn to do to increase your brain power is to learn how to pay better attention. Attention is the gateway to our memory and when we have problems remembering things, it is often because we were not paying attention when we had the experience in the first place. Some suggestions for improving your skills at paying attention include:

- Look around. At any time, look around yourself (up and down, left and right, and behind you) and notice what you see. Most of the time we focus only on what is in front of us. By looking around, you will improve your attention skills by not taking your surroundings for granted. You can do this at any time (walking, while being a passenger in a vehicle, sitting in a room, etc.).

- Notice details. At any time, notice new and different details of a familiar environment. What can you perceive that is new?

- Use all your senses. At any time, notice what you can about your environment using all of your senses (sight, sound, touch, smell, taste). Typically we are very visually oriented and don't focus on our other senses.

DRAGON GATE ATTENTION EXERCISE

- Find a comfortable place to sit. This can be inside or outside, but you should make sure that there are no major distractions such as noise, weather, etc.

- Close your eyes and take 3 deep breaths.

- With your eyes closed, use your sense of smell to take in your surroundings. What do you smell? Is there food cooking? Are there flowers nearby? Are you wearing perfume or cologne? Spend 1 to 2 minutes paying attention using the sense of smell.

- With your eyes closed, use your sense of touch to take in your surroundings. What do you feel? What are you sitting on? Is it soft or hard? Is the temperature warm or cold? Spend 1 to 2 minutes paying attention using the sense of touch.

- With your eyes closed, use your sense of taste to take in your surroundings. What can you taste? Is there something in the air you are breathing? Can you still taste the remnants of a meal you ate? Spend 1 to 2 minutes paying attention using the sense of taste.

- With your eyes closed, use your sense of hearing to take in your surroundings. Are there birds chirping? A siren in the distance? An airplane high overhead? Spend 1 to 2 minutes paying attention using the sense of hearing.

- Now open your eyes and use your sense of sight to take in your surroundings. What do you see? Go beyond the obvious. Look into the nooks and crannies of your environment. Notice subtle changes in lighting and color. Spend 1 to 2 minutes paying attention using the sense of sight.

- You may return to the same location at a later time and do the same exercise again. Notice how you can continually find new sensory stimuli.

☯ Remember

Memory is a critical mental factor that enables us to retain what we learn and experience in order to grow. Yet, memory is also a cognitive ability that tends to suffer the most as we age. But it doesn't have to be that way. Studies have shown that elderly people can maintain the same level of recall as people in their so called "prime" by maintaining a healthy lifestyle and exercising their memories. Some keys to improved memory are paying attention (as noted above), associating memories with a network of memories, and practicing memory exercises (such as memorizing texts, lists, statistics, phone numbers, names, and so on).

Dragon Gate Sense Memory Exercise

1. Before you begin, choose an event in your recent past that you have a good memory of. It can be any event that has occurred.

2. Find a comfortable place to sit or lie down. This can be inside or outside, but you should make sure that there are no major distractions such as noise, weather, etc.

3. Close your eyes and take 3 deep breaths.

4. With your eyes closed, try to remember everything you can about your event using your sense of smell. What can you remember of how the event smelled? Were there flowers? Was someone wearing perfume? Was there food? Spend 1 to 2 minutes remembering your event using the sense of smell.

5. With your eyes closed, try to remember everything you can about your event using your sense of touch. What can you remember of what you physically felt at your event? Did you touch someone, something? Was the air cool or hot? Spend 1 to 2 minutes remembering your event using the sense of touch.

6. With your eyes closed, try to remember everything you can about your event using your sense of taste. Did you eat something? Did the air have a taste to it? Spend 1 to 2 minutes remembering your event using the sense of taste.

7. With your eyes closed, try to remember everything you can about your event using your sense of hearing. Was there music playing? Was someone talking? Was there traffic noise outside? Spend 1 to 2 minutes remembering your event using the sense of hearing.

8. With your eyes closed, try to remember everything you can about your event using your sense of sight. What did the

event look like? Go beyond the obvious details and seek out minor details you may think you didn't even notice. What was someone wearing? What was the pattern on the wall-paper? Spend 1 to 2 minutes remembering your event using the sense of sight.

9. You may use the same event at a later time and do the same exercise again. Notice how you can continually find new memories.

Change Things Up

A key ingredient you can use to develop your mental abilities is employing novelty to constantly create new challenges and experiences for yourself. These new experiences can create new associations between different parts of the brain. So you can easily boost your cognitive abilities by simply switching things up on yourself.

For instance, pick an activity you always do in the light and do it in the dark and vice versa. You can also practice this method by brushing your teeth with your other hand, walking backwards, taking new routes on your regular journeys, and preparing new foods that you have never cooked with before. It can make life more fun and interesting and stimulate your brain at the same time.

As a general rule, try to do something different every day, no matter how insignificant, and approach every day as a living experiment and learning opportunity.

> It's never too late to start. With a little effort, even people in their seventies and eighties can see dramatic improvements.
>
> —DENNIS FOTH, PH.D., UNIVERSITY OF ALBERTA

Fifth Gate:
The Five Elements of Life

Understanding and Using the
Taoist Five Elements of Life

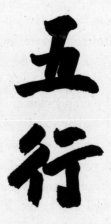

Five Elements

If your actions follow the Tao, you will progress. If your actions stray from the Tao, your progress will be halted.

—Shui-ch'ing Tzu, *Cultivating Stillness*

Please take a moment now before you begin this chapter to practice this brief and simple exercise. It will help you to maximize
your enjoyment of the chapter.

Relax and close your eyes. Choose one of the five elements
(wood, fire, earth, metal, or water). Pick whichever one occurs to
you first. Now focus on that element and feel yourself becoming
that element. Do this for 2 to 3 minutes.

Now you are ready to begin.

The Five Elements

The Tao is that energy that has existed from the beginning when
there was neither structure nor differentiation. It is the source of
life in heaven and on earth. It creates and is all things.

—SHUI-CH'ING TZU

Dragon Gate Taoism adheres to the Chinese system of the five elements. These five elements—wood, fire, earth, metal, and water—
represent the five different forms of organic and inorganic matter in
the universe. They are also often referred to as five movements,
phases, or steps because they are a metaphorical way of describing
essential patterns in every aspect of life in this time and space (in
Taoism, everything is relative to the time and space in which you
find yourself). Taoists believe that these five elemental patterns relate to everything, and they have applied them to areas as diverse as
medicine, martial arts, food, geography, feng shui, and music.

According to Dragon Gate philosophy, the five elements are the
creative and controlling energies of our planet. These elements are

in a constant state of flux, and their interdependence and interactions explain the complex connection between humanity and the natural world. Every aspect of our bodies, our lives, and the world around us can be categorized into one of these five perpetually flowing and interacting elements. For instance, each element is associated with a specific organ within our body (liver, spleen, stomach, lungs, and heart), a direction in the world around us (east, west, north, south, and center) and a color (green, red, yellow, white, and blue).

The origin of the five elements is not known. Various accounts suggest that the five elements theory may date back to the late Western Zhou period (eleventh century B.C.–770 B.C.) though some mythological accounts place it much earlier and attribute the development of the five elements to Fu Hsi, the mythological founder of Chinese civilization who is said to have lived approximately five thousand years ago. It was during the Zhou period when the first organized theories of yin and yang and the five elements arose as part of the development of Chinese ideas on the origin of the universe and the earliest methods of astrology.

The five elements became an essential aspect of Chinese medical theory when they were made a key portion of *The Yellow Emperor's Classic of Internal Medicine* (written approximately two thousand years ago). This seminal work, which is considered the most important ancient text in Chinese medicine as well as a major book of Taoist theory and lifestyle, used the theory of five elements and yin-yang to explain the physiological functions, as well as the causes, diagnosis, treatment, and methods of preventing illness. As with the works of astrology, politics, and philosophy, the Yellow Emperor proposed that it was the harmonious interaction of the elements that was of prime importance. The five elements remain an integral part of Chinese medicine to this day.

During the Eastern Zhou period (770 B.C.–256 B.C.), an era also designated as the period of the Hundred Schools of Thought when multiple Chinese philosophical traditions, including Confucianism, Mohism, Taoism, and Legalism, first appeared, the five elements theory was further developed and refined. (Confucianism, based on the teachings of Confucius, held that cultivation of morality and virtue were at the heart of creating a good society. Mohism, derived from the teachings of Mo Tzu, promoted a theory of society that embraced simplicity, morality, and merit. Legalism was based on the idea that people need to be controlled using laws in order to prevent chaos.) Tsou-Yen, a philosopher who lived in the fourth century B.C., wrote a treatise on cosmogony in which the five elements play an important part.

The five elements also figure prominently in *The Great Plan*, an ancient manifesto on the art of good government that theorizes that all good or bad fortune arises from the harmonious or inharmonious relationship among the five elements in a given situation. For instance, *The Great Plan* cites the following tale: "In olden times K'wan dammed up the inundating waters and so disarranged the five elements. The Emperor of Heaven was aroused to anger and would not give him the nine divisions of the Great Plan. In this way the several relations of society were disturbed, and for punishment he was kept in prison until he died."

Over the years, the role of the five element philosophy has been adapted to fit every aspect of life.

The Cycles of the Five Elements

Flow with whatever may happen and let your mind be free. Stay
centered by accepting whatever you are doing. This is the ultimate.

—CHUANG TZU

The five elements are largely defined by the relationships among the
elements. In other words, each of the elements interacts with the
other elements by helping to create, subdue, foster, or hinder them.
This is meant to parallel the patterns we see in life. Everything in
the world experiences a cycle marked by a beginning, development,
and ultimately decline. Likewise, in our lives, we see various paths
to success and failure, prosperity and poverty, health and illness,
wisdom and ignorance, etc.

In the cycle of the five elements, each of the elements has the
property of generating or "being generated." This cycle was described clearly in the second century A.D. by Liu An, a Chinese no-
bleman and scholar who authored *The Huainan Philosophers*, which
is one of the essential texts of Taoism. He wrote:

"By wood can be produced fire, by fire can be produced earth [that is,
fire burns wood, which turns to soil]; from earth can be produced
metal [for example, by mining]; from metal can be produced water
[that is, metal can be changed through heat to a liquid state]; from
water can be produced wood [that is, water feeds plants]. When fire
heats metal, it makes it liquid. When water destroys fire it operates
adversely upon the very element by which it is produced. Fire produces earth, yet earth counteracts water. No one can do anything
against these phenomena, for the power that causes the five elements
to counteract each other is according to the natural dispensation of

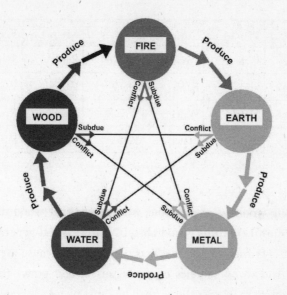

heaven and earth. Large quantities prevail over small quantities, hence water conquers fire. Spirituality prevails over materiality, the non-substance over substance, thus fire conquers metal; hardness conquers softness, hence metal conquers wood; density is superior to incoherence, therefore, wood conquers earth; solidity conquers insolidity, therefore earth conquers water."

There are two main phases in the five element cycle, a generating or creating phase and an overcoming or destructive phase. This pattern is shown in the figure below. The clockwise sequence on the circle represents the nourishing cycle or the mother-son cycle. In other words, each element is parent to the next element. The clockwise sequence depicted by the pentagon represents the regulating or destructive cycle.

In this way, each element has a direct relationship with each of the other four elements as shown in the following chart:

ELEMENT	WOOD	FIRE	EARTH	METAL	WATER
Dissolves	Water	Wood	Fire	Earth	Metal
Generates	Fire	Earth	Metal	Water	Wood
Conflicts	Metal	Water	Wood	Fire	Earth
Subdues	Earth	Metal	Water	Wood	Fire

Taking wood, as an example, you can see that wood dissolves water—in other words, wood absorbs water. Wood generates fire when it is burned. Wood conflicts with metal, because metal cuts wood. And wood subdues earth, because wood grows from the earth and its roots part the earth. The same phases operate on the other elements as well.

APPLYING THE FIVE ELEMENTS TO YOUR LIFE

Now that you understand what the five elements are and how they interact you may naturally be wondering how to best apply this knowledge to your own life. The key to using the five elements, as with all Taoist practice, is knowing how to maintain the correct balance. As the Chinese medical classic the *Leijing tuyi* (Illustrated Commentary for the Classic of Internal Medicine) states, "If there is no generation, then there is no growth and development. If there is no restriction, then endless growth and development will become harmful."

No doubt you can view your own life and see areas that are doing just fine, areas that require nourishment, and areas that are out of control. By using the balancing, nourishing, and subduing formulas of the five elements you may be able to more accurately view your own situation and devise the best strategies for balancing the elements in your own life. As you learn to better understand which element you are dealing with in any given situation and how to complement it or transform it, you gain the ability to successfully adapt to and influence the underlying forces of your physical reality.

Applying the idea of the five elements on a metaphorical level is an extremely powerful idea and allows the Dragon Gate practitioner to utilize these concepts. As with every aspect of Dragon Gate practice, the purpose is to expand your consciousness and open your reality to new ideas and ways of expressing all that you are and all that you hope to become. It is not a method for creating artificial limitations and fears that block you into a fixed mode of looking at the world.

To give you a sense of how the Chinese philosophers have attempted to apply five element theory to the world around us, here is a chart that outlines some of the basic phenomena associated with each element.

Using the chart on page 102 as a guide, you can view different areas of your life and determine which element represents it. For instance, if you are having health issues with your respiratory system, you can see that the respiratory system is part of the metal element. So to strengthen that body system you can eat spicy food (e.g., ginger), wear more metal jewelry, put metal artwork around your house, use more white coloring in clothing and design, etc.

One of the very best ways to gain access to the power of the five elements is through the use of the Dragon Gate five element exercises (and the five celestial guardians, which will be explained in the

The Five Elements and Their Associated Phenomena

ELEMENT	WOOD	FIRE	EARTH	METAL	WATER
Energy Pattern	Generating	Expanding	Stabilizing	Contracting	Flowing
Yin/Yang Phase	New Yang	Full Yang	Yin-Yang Balance	New Yin	Full Yin
Development	Sprouting	Blooming	Ripening	Withering	Dormancy
Direction	East	South	Center	West	North
Color	Green	Red	Yellow	White	Dark Blue/ Black
Season	Spring	Summer	Seasonal Transition	Autumn	Winter
Climate	Wind	Heat	Damp	Dry	Cold
Yang Organ	Gall Bladder	Small Intestine	Stomach	Large Intestine	Bladder
Yin Organ	Liver	Heart	Spleen	Lung	Kidney
Sense Organ	Eyes	Tongue	Mouth	Nose	Ears
Body Tissue	Sinews	Blood Vessels	Muscles	Skin	Bone
Body System	Metabolism/ Hormone	Cardiovascular/ Brain	Digestion	Respiratory/ Immune	Reproductive/ Urinary
Emotion	Anger	Joy/Surprise	Worry/ Concern	Sadness/ Grief	Fear
Taste	Sour	Bitter	Sweet	Spicy/ Pungent	Salty
Planet	Jupiter	Mars	Saturn	Venus	Mercury

next chapter). These simple but very powerful exercises are detailed below. You can practice these to stimulate each of the five elements in your life. So, using the respiratory example cited above, you could do the metal exercises and visualization to strengthen your respiratory system.

With a little dedicated practice of these exercises you will find yourself becoming more attuned to the five elements and how they play a role in your life.

Five Element Exercises

The following exercises are specifically designed to activate, energize, and work with the energy associated with each corresponding element using a combination of chi development movements and nature practices. These practices are also excellent for promoting positive energy and health for the organs associated with each element. You may combine the chi gung (energy exercise) portion and the nature portion, or you may do each one separately.

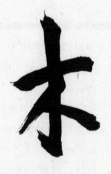

As it acts in the world, the Tao is like the
    bending of a tree.
The top is bent downward; the bottom
    is bent up.
It adjusts excess and deficiency so that there
    is perfect balance.

               —LAO TZU

Wood

On a physical level, wood represents all plant life on earth. On a metaphorical level, the wood element represents flexibility, creativity, and growth.

WOOD ELEMENT EXERCISES

🌓 *Nature Practice*

1. If you have access to the outdoors, find a tree that you would like to practice with. This can be a tree in your backyard or a tree that you have never seen before in a park or forest. The size of the tree does not matter. Simply seek out a tree that appeals to you. If you live somewhere where you do not have access to trees, you may use a house plant or a photo of a tree.

2. Find a comfortable place to stand or sit near your tree. Make sure that there are no major distractions such as noise, weather, etc. You may stand or sit facing the tree or with your back to the tree. If it is a small tree or plant you can even partially encircle it with your arms. The main point is to be comfortable and feel at ease.

3. Close your eyes and take 3 nice, deep breaths. Then spend a few moments contemplating the essence and energy of the tree. You may also touch the tree by placing your palms on the trunk and feeling its energy. When you do this, feel a vortex of energy in the center of your palms that interacts with the energy of the tree. Sense its roots going deep into the ground and pulling up nutrients from the soil. (If you are using a house plant, you can touch a leaf and if you are

using a photograph, you can touch the photo. While these may require a bit more imagination, you can obtain similar results to being in nature.)

4. Spend 3 to 5 minutes in this practice (you may extend the time as you wish).

5. To conclude, if you have extended your hands, close the energy vortex in your palms and bring your arms to your sides. Then bring the energy you have gathered to your dantian (the energy center at your navel) and take 3 deep breaths.

6. In future you may return to the same tree or select a different tree.

☯ *Chi Gung Practice*

This practice is ideally done in the morning soon after waking or in the evening before bed. However, if those times are not convenient, you can do this exercise whenever it is best for you.

1. Face east and stand with your feet shoulder-width apart. (If you do not know which direction is east, simply face in the direction that most appeals to you.)

2. Keeping your head straight, look ahead, smile, and allow your arms to hang down freely at your sides keeping your hands in a "sword fist" where your index and middle fingers are extended and the three remaining fingers are folded in a soft fist.

3. Keeping your hands in the "sword fist" raise them toward your chest, bending at the elbows and palms facing up. While you do this, breathe in deeply while pulling in your abdomen and tightening the muscles around your perineum (anus).

4. Next you are going to breathe out in combination with the following movements: without moving your feet, rotate your torso slowly to your left till you can turn no further while simultaneously extending your right arm in front of you at a 45-degree angle and extending your left arm down in back at a 45-degree angle to your right (both arms should be lined up on the same plane, your bottom palm should face up and your top palm should face down). As you do this, your eyes follow your right middle-finger tip and you slowly make the sound "shhhhh" while relaxing the muscles around perineum and those in abdomen. (The sound "shhhhh" should be like air rushing out of a punctured tire.)

5. Return to your starting position by turning the torso back to the right and slowly lowering your arms while breathing naturally.

6. Keeping your hands in the "sword fist" raise them toward your chest, bending at the elbows, palms facing up. While you do this, breathe in deeply while pulling in your abdomen and tightening the muscles around your perineum (anus).

7. Next you are going to breathe out in combination with the following movements: without moving your feet, rotate your torso slowly to your right till you can turn no further while simultaneously extending your left arm in front of you at a 45-degree angle and extending your right arm down in back at a 45-degree angle (both arms should be lined up on the same plane and both palms should face up). As you do this, your eyes follow your left middle-finger tip and you slowly make the sound "shhhhh" while relaxing the muscles around perineum and those in abdomen.

8. Repeat this process 7 times for a total of 8 circuits.

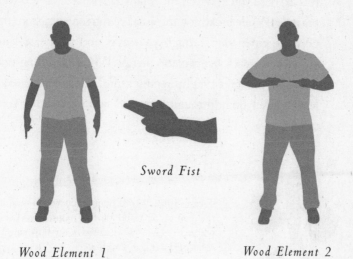

Sword Fist

Wood Element 1   Wood Element 2

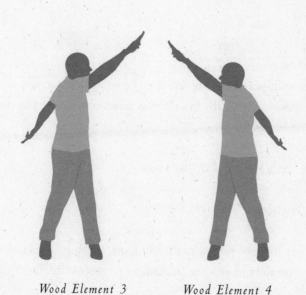

Wood Element 3   Wood Element 4

9. Additional visualization: once you are comfortable doing this exercise you may add the following visualization to your practice. While breathing in, visualize a green light from the universe enter you through your eyes and permeate your entire body with benevolent energy. While breathing out, visualize the green light representing benevolent energy leaving your body through your eyes and permeating your universe.

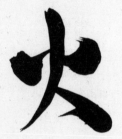

Fire

Taoism is the way of man's cooperation with the course or trend of the natural world, whose principles we discover in the flow patterns of water, gas, and fire.

—ALAN WATTS

On a physical level, fire represents combustion and all gases. On a metaphorical level, the fire element represents energy and passion.

FIRE ELEMENT EXERCISES

☯ *Nature Practice*

1. If you have access to the outdoors, for this practice you may use the sun or a fire (remember never to stare directly at the

sun). If you are practicing indoors, you may use a fire in a fireplace or a candle.

2. Find a comfortable place to stand or sit where you have a clear view of your source of "fire." Make sure that there are no major distractions such as noise, weather, etc. The main point is to be comfortable and feel at ease.

3. Close your eyes and take 3 deep breaths. Then spend a few moments contemplating and feeling the essence and energy of the fire. You may extend your palms toward the fire. If you are using the sun, feel how it is the source of all life on earth. If you are using another source of flame, feel its warmth and energy. When you do this, feel a vortex of energy in the center of your palms that interacts with the energy of the fire.

4. Spend 3 to 5 minutes in this practice (you may extend the time as you wish).

5. To conclude, if you have extended your hands, close the energy vortex in your palms and bring your arms to your sides. Then bring the energy you have gathered to your dantian and take 3 very deep breaths.

☯ Chi Gung Practice

1. This practice is ideally done in the morning soon after waking or in the evening before bed. However, if those times are not convenient, you can do this exercise whenever it is best for you.

2. Face south and stand with your feet shoulder-width apart. If you do not know which direction is south, simply face in

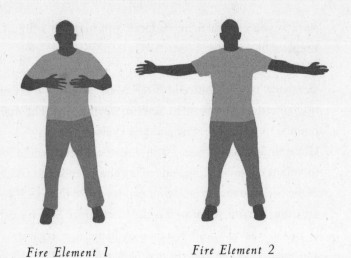

Fire Element 1   *Fire Element 2*

the direction that most appeals to you. (This exercise can also be done lying down.)

3. Keeping your head straight, look ahead and smile. Now place your palms on your chest so that the tips of your middle fingers touch each other lightly directly in the center of your chest at the midpoint between your nipples. (Keep your shoulders relaxed.)

4. Slowly open your arms wide until they are in line with your chest (not in front and not behind your chest). While you do this, breathe in deeply through your nose while pulling in your abdomen and tightening the muscles around your perineum (anus).

5. Next you are going to breathe out in combination with the following movements: slowly move both hands back to their original position over your chest. As you do this, slowly make the sound "hhhhhaaaaaa" while relaxing the muscles

around the perineum and the abdomen. (The "hhhhhaaaaaa" sound is like breathing out audibly.)

6. Repeat this process 6 times for a total of 7 circuits.

7. Additional visualization: Once you are comfortable doing this exercise you may add the following visualization to your practice. While breathing in, visualize a red light from the universe enter you through your mouth and permeate your entire body with joyful energy. While breathing out, visualize the red light representing joyful energy leaving your body through your mouth and permeating your universe.

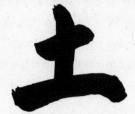

Man follows the earth.
Earth follows the universe.
The universe follows the Tao.

—LAO TZU

Earth

On a physical level, earth represents soil, rocks, clay, stone, etc. On a metaphorical level, the earth element represents stability, permanence, and a medium for growth.

EARTH ELEMENT EXERCISES

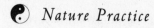 *Nature Practice*

1. If you have access to the outdoors, find a place where you have contact with the earth. If you are practicing indoors, you may use a plant or a small plate of soil.

2. Find a comfortable place to stand or sit where you have a clear view of your source of "earth." Make sure that there are no major distractions such as noise, weather, etc. The main point is to be comfortable and feel at ease. If you are outside and the conditions are appropriate, it is best if you can remove your shoes and socks and stand or sit so that your feet come into direct contact with the ground.

3. Close your eyes and take 3 deep breaths. Then spend a few moments contemplating and feeling the essence and energy of the earth. Feel how the earth is the mother from which your life sprang—how you are part of the earth. You may extend your palms toward the earth. When you do this, feel a vortex of energy in the center of your palms that interacts with the energy of the earth. If you are standing, feel a vortex of energy in the bottom of your feet that interacts with the energy of the earth.

4. Spend 3 to 5 minutes in this practice (you may extend the time as you wish).

5. To conclude, if you have extended your hands, close the energy vortex in your palms and bring your arms to your sides. Then bring the energy you have gathered to your dantian and take 3 very deep breaths.

☯ Chi Gung Practice

1. This practice is ideally done in the morning soon after waking or in the evening before bed. However, if those times are not convenient, you can do this exercise whenever it is best for you.

2. If you are a person who prefers cold over heat, face northeast. If you are a person who prefers heat over cold face southwest. (If you do not know which direction is northeast/southwest, simply face in the direction that most appeals to you.)

3. Keeping your head straight, look ahead and smile. Allow your arms to hang relaxed by your sides.

4. Slowly turn your palms so they face up and move them in front of your body so the fingers of both hands point at each other. Now slowly raise both hands until they reach the level of your armpits. While you do this, breathe in deeply through your nose while pulling in your abdomen and tightening the muscles around your perineum (anus).

5. Next you are going to breathe out in combination with the following movements: slowly turn your palms over so they face down and push down until your arms are fully extended. As you do this, slowly make the sound "oooohng" (which sounds like the "aum" mantra) while relaxing the muscles around the perineum and the abdomen.

6. Repeat this process 8 times for a total of 9 circuits.

7. Additional visualization: Once you are comfortable doing this exercise you may add the following visualization to your practice. While breathing in, visualize a yellow light from the universe enter you through your navel and permeate your entire body with trust energy. While breathing out, visualize the yellow light representing trust energy leaving your body through your navel and permeating your universe.

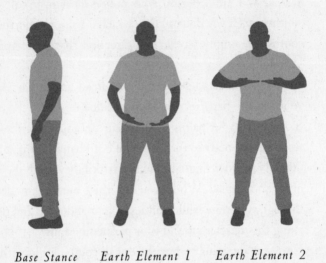

Base Stance   *Earth Element 1*   *Earth Element 2*

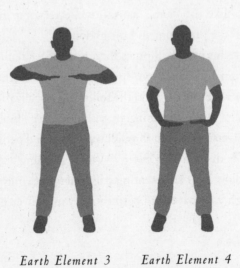

Earth Element 3   *Earth Element 4*

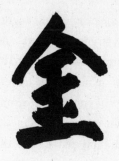

A good cook goes through a knife in a year,
Because he cuts.
An average cook goes through a knife in a
        month,
Because he hacks.

—CHUANG TZU

Metal

On a physical level, metal represents every kind of metal and mineral. On a metaphorical level, the metal element represents a conductor of energy, connection, and strength.

METAL ELEMENT EXERCISES

Nature Practice

1. If you find yourself in the fortunate position of having access to a natural source of metal ore in a rock face, or in an area where metals occur naturally, then definitely use that. Otherwise find a piece of metal that has particular significance for you. Gold is preferable, but any metal will work.

2. Find a comfortable place to stand or sit where you have a clear view of your source of "metal." Make sure that there are no major distractions such as noise, weather, etc. The main point is to be comfortable and feel at ease.

3. Close your eyes and take 3 deep breaths. Then spend a few

moments contemplating and feeling the essence and energy of the metal. Feel the malleability and strength of metal and feel how the metal element courses through your body in the form of minerals. You may extend your palms toward the metal. When you do this, feel a vortex of energy in the center of your palms that interacts with the energy of the metal.

4. Spend 3 to 5 minutes in this practice (you may extend the time as you wish).

5. To conclude, if you have extended your hands, close the energy vortex in your palms and bring your arms to your sides. Then bring the energy you have gathered to your dantian and take 3 deep breaths.

☯ Chi Gung Practice

1. This practice is ideally done in the morning soon after waking or in the evening before bed. However, if those times are not convenient, you can do this exercise whenever it is best for you.

2. Face west with your feet shoulder-width apart. If you do not know which direction is west, simply face in the direction that most appeals to you.

3. Keeping your head straight, look ahead and smile. Allow your arms to hang relaxed by your sides.

4. Slowly turn your palms so they face up and slowly raise both hands (keeping them at your sides) until they reach the level of your armpits. While you do this, breathe in deeply through your nose while pulling in your abdomen and tightening the muscles around your perineum (anus).

5. Next you are going to breathe out in combination with the following movements: make a tiger fist (fingers bent, but not closed into a full fist), and then extend your arms slowly with your fists facing each other on an angle. Push your fists forward until your arms are fully extended (once your arms are extended the palms of your hands should be facing out). As you do this, slowly make the sound "sssiiii" (which sounds something like a snake hiss) while relaxing the muscles around the perineum and the abdomen. This is the only five element exercise where you should use some force (a moderate level).

6. Then, open your hands and swing your arms back to your sides (where your arms were when you started to breathe out) as though you are swimming the breast stroke. While you do this, breathe in deeply through your nose while pulling in your abdomen and tightening the muscles around your perineum (anus).

7. Repeat this process 8 times for a total of 9 circuits.

8. Additional visualization: Once you are comfortable doing this exercise you may add the following visualization to your practice. While breathing in, visualize a white light from the universe enter you through your nose and permeate your entire body with brilliance energy. While breathing out, visualize the white light representing brilliance energy leaving your body through your nose and permeating your universe.

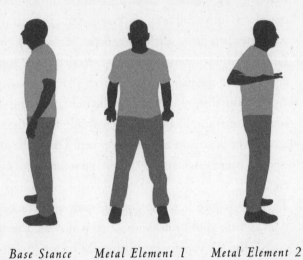

Base Stance   *Metal Element 1*   *Metal Element 2*

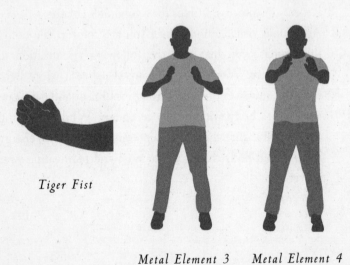

Tiger Fist

Metal Element 3   *Metal Element 4*

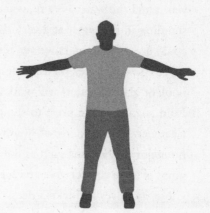

Metal Element 5   *Metal Element 6*

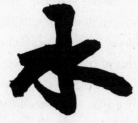

Under heaven nothing is more soft and
   yielding than water.
Yet for attacking the solid and strong,
   nothing is better. It has no equal.

— LAO TZU

Water

On a physical level, water represents every kind of liquid. On a metaphorical level, the water element represents communication, wealth, and flow.

WATER ELEMENT EXERCISES

☯ *Nature Practice*

1. For this exercise, it is best to use flowing water. Outside this would be a river, a stream, or the ocean. (If the weather is

warm and the water is calm, you can do this exercise while standing in the water at a very shallow depth.) Inside, you could use a fountain. However, if you do not have ready access to flowing water, then standing water (a lake, swimming pool, or glass of water) will work as well.

2. Find a comfortable place to stand or sit where you have a clear view of your source of "water." Make sure that there are no major distractions such as noise, weather, etc. The main point is to be comfortable and feel at ease.

3. Close your eyes and take 3 deep breaths. Then spend a few moments contemplating and feeling the essence of the water. Contemplate the flowing energy of water, how water can wear down rocks into sand. Feel how water makes up over 80 percent of your body and the essential nature of water in the process of life. You may extend your palms toward the water. When you do this, feel a vortex of energy in the center of your palms that interacts with the energy of the metal.

4. Spend 3 to 5 minutes in this practice (you may extend the time as you wish).

5. To conclude, if you have extended your hands, close the energy vortex in your palms and bring your arms to your sides. Then bring the energy you have gathered to your dantian and take 3 deep breaths.

☯ Chi Gung Practice

1. This practice is ideally done in the morning soon after waking or in the evening before bed. However, if those times are not convenient, you can do this exercise whenever it is best for you.

2. Face north with your feet shoulder-width apart. (If you do not know which direction is north, simply face in the direction that most appeals to you.)

3. Keeping your head straight, look ahead and smile. Allow your arms to hang relaxed by your sides.

4. Rub your palms together briskly (generating some friction heat) in front of your abdomen 36 times. Then cover your navel with both hands. For women, place the left hand over the right hand. For men, place the right hand over the left hand.

5. Bend your body backward at the waist about 15 degrees. While you do this, breathe in deeply while pulling in your abdomen and tightening the muscles around your perineum (anus).

6. Next you are going to breathe out in combination with the following movements: bend your torso forward at the waist about 45 degrees, pressing your hands lightly on your abdomen at the navel. As you do this, slowly make the sound "ohhhh" while relaxing the muscles around the perineum and the abdomen.

7. Repeat this process 2 times for a total of 3 circuits.

8. Additional visualization: Once you are comfortable doing this exercise you may add the following visualization to your practice. While breathing in, visualize a dark blue light from the universe enter you through your ears and permeate your entire body with peace energy. While breathing out, visualize the dark blue light representing peace energy leaving your body through your ears and permeating your universe.

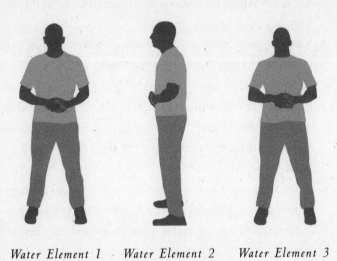

Water Element 1   Water Element 2   Water Element 3

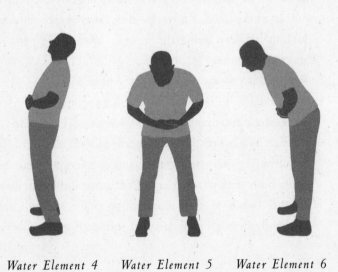

Water Element 4   Water Element 5   Water Element 6

Sixth Gate:
Taoist Shamanism
and Dream Yoga

DRAGON GATE DREAM YOGA PRACTICE

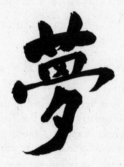

Dream

I dreamed I was a butterfly, flying in the sky; then I awoke. Now I wonder, am I a man who dreamt of being a butterfly, or am I a butterfly dreaming that I am a man?

—CHUANG TZU

Please take a moment now before you begin this chapter to practice this brief and simple exercise. It will help you to maximize your enjoyment of the chapter.

Close your eyes and take a few moments to relax. Then think about an event that happened in your life today as though it was part of a dream. Do not imagine that it was a dream—think about it exactly as you would if the experiences you had were part of a dream.

Now you are ready to begin.

The Shamanic Roots of Taoism

Mystics have never been very interested in theology. Mystics are interested in direct experience. And the Taoists, being mystics, were the only great group of ancient Chinese people who seriously studied nature. They were interested in its principles from the beginning, and their books are full of analogies between the Taoist way of life and the behavior of natural forces seen in water, wind, or plants and rocks.

—ALAN WATTS

Taoism's origins, like those of many other spiritual philosophies and belief systems, can be traced back to shamanic practices from the earliest tribal civilizations. The word *shaman* comes from the Tungusic language of a tribe in Siberia (who used the word *saman*), the study of which initiated Western interest into the practice of shamanism.

A shaman is a man or a woman who "journeys" from our "ordinary" reality into a "non-ordinary" reality, typically in an altered state of consciousness brought about through drumming, meditation, or the ingestion of psychoactive plants. In these other states of consciousness, or "non-ordinary" reality, the shaman is able to travel to far-off locations outside of time and space and establish relationships with spirits and other non-human entities. He or she can then bring back information that is useful for the community in this reality.

Shamanic practices are mainly found in tribal cultures and the word *shaman* is often used as a synonym for medicine man or woman. Most of the world's religions have grown out of shamanic practices and their traces can still be seen in the rituals and beliefs, whether it's a Taoist using herbal medicine or a Catholic eating the body of Christ in the Eucharist.

While there are many variations of shamanism throughout the world there are unifying themes, which include:

- The belief that all things in our world have consciousness.
- Communication with spirits (non-human forms of consciousness). These spirits can become guides or helpers. They can also be the source of problems or illnesses experienced in our ordinary reality.
- Journeying into other realms of consciousness.
- Healing. This can be through the use of herbs and other elements that are found in our reality, as well as efforts undertaken on the ill person's behalf in the spirit world.
- Divination, or predicting the future.
- A deep respect for, and in some cases worship of, nature.

A key element of shamanic practice is the idea that the work being done in the spirit world is specifically designed to make a practical difference in our physical world.

Being one with Nature, he is in accord with the Tao.
Being in accord with the Tao, he is everlasting.

—Lao Tzu

The Chinese word for shaman, or *wu*, was first recorded during the Shang dynasty (1600 B.C.–1046 B.C.), but it is believed that these practices date back to the very origins of Chinese culture. In fact, many of the stories surrounding Fu Hsi, the mythical founder of Chinese civilization (approximately five thousand years ago) have a distinctly shamanic feel to them. For instance, Fu Hsi is considered the creator of the Yi Jing (I Ching), or Book of Changes, the basis of all Chinese philosophy. According to the legend, he discovered the Yi Jing in the arrangement of markings on the back of a turtle that emerged from a river. This is a classic shamanic tale that marries nature and divination with the result being the attainment of profound knowledge.

In the historical documents that remain, the wu (shamans) are portrayed as masters of many magical talents including exorcism, healing, divination, and rainmaking. They were also known to enter trance states and journey into the spirit world to gather information. The ancient Chinese emperors employed these shamans to assist them in choosing the appropriate course of action and maintaining their power.

There is even a record of an ancient Chinese hallucinogen, yun-shih (*Caesalpinia sepiaria*) a shrubby vine believed to possess medical and magical properties. The earliest Chinese herbal manual states that the yun-shih flowers "contain occult powers" that allowed "one to see spirits." The book also claimed that the flowers "produce levitation of the body and promote communication with the spirits."

With the rise of Confucianism and Buddhism, the wu practice slowly fell out of favor. Shamans were persecuted, like witches in the West, and ultimately their practices were completely banned. However, they continued their rituals and training in secret and became known as magicians, wizards, and sorcerers. As time went on and shamanism receded from Chinese culture, the shaman's duties were largely taken over by Taoists. A key to the rapid rise of Taoism as a state-backed philosophy/religion is that it repeatedly sought to adopt the beliefs of other philosophies and religions, including Buddhism, Confucianism, and the shamanic folk traditions that preceded them all.

At their core, both shamanism and Taoism work on developing, channeling, and directing energies within their practitioners and in the world around them. To this day, these ideas can be seen throughout Taoism in practices ranging from healing, divination, and astrology to spirit travel and the use of talismans. It is also at the heart of feng shui (literally "wind and water"), the Taoist art of placement, which guides practitioners on the best way to create a positive and nurturing environment. Of course most Taoist rituals as well as chi gung (energy exercises) are designed to enable the practitioner to live in harmony with nature. Shamanic influences can also be seen clearly in Taoist alchemy, sexual yoga, and the dream yoga described in this chapter.

The result of Taoism's multiple influences was that it developed as both a philosophy of spontaneity and naturalism and a folk religion that specialized in rituals and techniques for achieving immortality. But at its core, the Tao is a path to the ideal life by living in harmony with nature—an inherently shamanic idea.

Eventually, from its shamanic roots, Taoism rose to become, for many centuries, the official state religion of China. It also formed the foundation of most Chinese art, traditional Chinese medicine such as acupuncture and herbalism, Chinese astrology and divination, meditative martial arts such as tai chi, and the esoteric alchemical practices such as sexual and dream yoga.

Dragon Gate Dream Yoga

Some day comes the great awakening when we realize that this life is no more than a dream. Yet the foolish go on thinking they are awake.
Surveying the panorama of life with such clarity, they call this one a prince and that one a peasant. What delusion!
The great Confucius and you are both a dream.
And I, who say all this is a dream, I, too, am a dream.
What mystery this vision contains!

—CHUANG TZU

Among the safest, most enjoyable, and easiest to learn and access shamanic practices in Taoism is dream yoga. *Yoga* is a Sanskrit word that means "union," or more specifically "union with the divine." However, the term *yoga* has been adopted now by many traditions as a shorthand to describe a spiritual practice. A "dream" yoga is one that harnesses the power of the dream and sleep states to awaken the consciousness. The idea behind dream yoga is simple. We spend approximately one third of our lives sleeping. So dream yoga gives us the opportunity to use that time as part of our practice.

Most of the esoteric traditions including Hinduism, Tibetan Buddhism, and Sufism as well as indigenous shamanic cultures have some type of dream yoga practice. But all cultures throughout the world are known to place importance on the power of dreams to access information that is typically hidden from our normal, waking consciousness. This can be seen in works ranging from the Bible to the writings of Freud and Jung.

In the West, dream yoga has come to be known as lucid dreaming, astral projection, or out-of-body experiences and the practitioners are sometimes known as oneironauts that comes from the Greek word *oneiros*, which means "dream." A lucid dream is one in which the practitioner becomes aware that he or she is dreaming while dreaming. In other words, the lucid dreamer can act deliberately in the dream state to do whatever he or she wants without the constraints of normal, physical reality.

According to studies, a majority of people have experienced a lucid dream—a dream in which they became aware that they were dreaming. A much smaller percentage, approximately 20 percent, reports having a lucid dream once a month or more. Among this percentage, active meditators report having the highest number of lucid dreams.

Aside from the obvious fun people can have if they become lucid in a dream—the ability to do anything you can think of certainly creates a lot of possibilities for wish fulfillment—learning to awaken within a dream offers many other benefits. These include increased energy, problem solving, enhancing our creativity, gaining insight into the death process, and cultivating our intuition. But perhaps the greatest spiritual benefit lies in helping the practitioner wake up to the dream-like nature of all experience, which is key to creating a magical Taoist reality.

Sleeping

If one advances confidently in the direction of one's dreams, and
endeavors to live the life which one has imagined, one will meet
with a success unexpected in common hours.

—HENRY DAVID THOREAU

Sleep research is a relatively young field. It became possible with the
invention of the electroencephalograph and other technologies that
allowed scientists to monitor brain activity and other functions that
had previously been hidden. Before people began studying sleep,
it was generally believed that most brain activity stopped during
sleep. The current science holds that we pass through four (or five,
depending on your classification system) stages of sleep every night,
each of which displays different brain wave patterns. The four
stages are further subdivided into two main types of sleep, which
are non–rapid eye movement (NREM), also known as quiet sleep,
and rapid eye movement (REM), also known as active sleep, during
which we dream.

Stage 1, sometimes known as hypnagogic sleep, is the beginning
of the sleep cycle. It is a relatively light stage of sleep that is essentially a transition between wakefulness and sleep. In Stage 1, the
brain transitions from producing beta waves to much slower alpha
waves. This period of sleep typically lasts only a short time. In this
stage, the eyes move slowly, muscle activity slows, and people often
experience unusual and extremely vivid sensations known as hypnagogic hallucinations.

Stage 2, or ordinary sleep, is when the brain begins to produce
bursts of rapid, rhythmic brain wave activity known as sleep spin-

dles. Body temperature decreases and heart rate slows. This stage occupies 45 to 55 percent of total sleep in adults.

Stage 3, or the deep sleep state, is one in which slow delta brain waves emerge. Stage 3 is where deep sleep phenomena such as sleepwalking and sleep-talking usually occur.

Stage 4, known as rapid eye movement (REM) sleep, is where it is believed that most dreaming occurs. During REM sleep, the eyes move rapidly and the body experiences an increase in respiration rate and brain activity. The waveform of REM sleep is similar to the waking state, but while the brain and other body systems are more active, muscles are more relaxed, which is why researchers initially called it "paradoxical sleep." It is believed that the body paralysis that accompanies dreaming protects us from injuring ourselves by physically acting out scenes that we are dreaming.

A complete sleep cycle takes an average of 90 to 110 minutes, during which time you move through these various stages, not necessarily in sequence. The first sleep cycles each night have relatively short REM sleep, but each cycle becomes longer, so as sleep progresses REM periods can last up to an hour. Most people experience three to five intervals of REM sleep each night. Infants spend almost 50 percent of their time in REM sleep while adults spend about 20 to 25 percent in REM. As we age, we tend to spend progressively less time in REM.

Developing Your Dream Practice

What is life? An illusion, a fiction, a passing shadow . . . for all of
life's a dream and dreams themselves are only part of dreaming.

—Pedro Calderón de la Barca,
seventeenth-century Spanish writer

Dragon Gate dream practice, sometimes called true dreaming,
dream wandering, or night practice, uses energy work and shamanic
techniques along with traditional dream yoga. The dream state can
then be used as a tool for energy development and enlightenment,
while the dreams themselves can become a source of spiritual direction or guidance.

There are several levels to dream practice. The prerequisite for
doing dream yoga is to establish healthy sleep patterns. You can do
this by following the six keys to a healthy life outlined in Chapter
2. As long as your sleep is healthy you are ready to begin Dragon
Gate dream yoga.

Life Is a Dream

How can you be certain that your whole life is not a dream?

—René Descartes

The essence of a lucid dream is recognizing that you are dreaming
during the dream. The first step in this process is to begin looking
at your normal waking reality as though it too is a dream. A basic
principle of Dragon Gate Taoism is that life is a dream of our own
creation. Dream yoga, then, is meant to help us wake up from this
dream in order to experience life completely.

So the very first exercise is to go about your daily activities reminding yourself that everything you are experiencing is a dream. How can you know for sure that what you are experiencing is not a dream?

As you go through your day, try to think of everything you experience, everyone you meet, everywhere you go as being part of a dream. This applies to everything from thinking of your physical possessions as dream possessions and your friends as dream friends, to thinking of the less tangible elements of your life such as problems or thoughts as dream problems and thoughts. Then, as you're lying in bed before going to sleep, review your day as though you were recounting a dream you had.

Another very simple practice along the same lines is doing what are known as "reality checks." This is where you constantly confirm whether you are dreaming or awake. You can do this by placing your hand on a wall and trying to move through the wall, or willing yourself to fly. Essentially, a reality check is attempting anything that you believe is impossible during normal waking reality as though you were in fact dreaming and it was completely possible.

The more you do these practices, the better the effect. Like any spiritual exercise, the longer and more consistently you practice it, the greater the benefit. Once the ideas captured by these methods become second nature, you will find yourself in a night-dream doing the same thing. In other words, you will notice that you are dreaming and then you will "wake up" in your dream and experience it consciously.

Here are two simple exercises you can do alone and with a friend to help spur your dream practice.

Dreaming Mirror Practice

1. Find a mirror that you can stand or sit in front of comfortably.
2. Take 3 deep breaths.
3. Spend a few moments looking at yourself in the mirror. Then, once you are completely relaxed, repeat to yourself, "You are dreaming."
4. Continue for 2 to 3 minutes.

Friends Dreaming Practice

1. Find a comfortable place where you and a friend can stand or sit facing each other. This can be inside or outside, but you should make sure that there are no major distractions such as noise, weather, etc. Choose who will go first.
2. Position yourselves so that your faces are 2 to 3 feet apart.
3. Take 3 deep breaths.
4. Spend a few moments looking at each other. Then, once you are completely relaxed, the person chosen to go first should say to their friend, slowly and clearly, "You are dreaming." The second person should wait a brief moment and then respond by saying, "You are dreaming."
5. Continue for 2 to 3 minutes.

It is very important to remember that believing that life is a dream does not mean that life is something trivial or meaningless. On the contrary, dream yoga is meant to empower your dreams—

both waking and sleeping—with greater conscious creatorhood. As with all Dragon Gate practice it is essential that you use the beliefs only to enhance your reality and not to denigrate it.

Transforming the Dream

All that we see is but a dream within a dream.
—EDGAR ALLAN POE

Once you begin experiencing lucid dreams you can then begin working on the process of transforming your dreams. To do this you need to take control of your dreams. You can do this in any number of ways that include willing yourself to fly, transforming objects in your dreams (such as shrinking or enlarging objects), and going to any location and meeting any person you wish.

As you proceed with this practice it is important to eliminate fear from your dream reality by recognizing that anything that occurs to you in a dream will not hurt you. You can start this process slowly by first creating a fire in your dream and then sticking your dream finger into the fire. Once you see that your finger doesn't burn, you can stick your arm and indeed your entire body into the fire. And as you get comfortable with this practice you can jump off buildings, skydive without a parachute, or do daredevil activities you would never undertake in waking reality.

The more advanced stages of this practice involve the realization that your dream body is as insubstantial as everything else in the dream. So in your dream you can alter the shape of your body, completely change your appearance, or even make your body disappear.

Recalling the Dream

Accurate knowledge about the signs which occur in dreams will
be found very valuable for all purposes.

—HIPPOCRATES

Another key element of dream practice is recalling the dream. After
all, think of everything you'll miss if you experience all these adventures during your sleep, but are unable to remember them when
you wake up. So the last thing you should do before going to sleep
is commit yourself to remembering the dreams you are about to
have. Then, the first thing you should do every morning when you
wake up is to do your best to recall the dreams you had the night
before.

It is a good idea to keep a dream journal by your bed that you
can write your dreams in if you wake up in the middle of the night
or the first thing in the morning. It is important to do this before
you even get out of bed. Dreams have an amazing way of disap-
pearing from your mind as soon as you get up and start going about
your day. By maintaining a journal, you can begin to recognize recurring images and themes, and it also helps in interpreting sym-
bolic content and meaning.

You will find that as you practice this more and more, you will
get better at it. Dragon Gate also has a dream recall exercise that is
part of the practice and that you can read about below.

Five Celestial Guardians

It is traditional in shamanism for the practitioner to cultivate various spirit guides who can assist the shaman in both the ordinary and non-ordinary reality. These guides can provide guidance, support, energy, and assistance in various ways. Dragon Gate Taoism has developed a group of five animal guides, based on the five elements and known as the "five celestial guardians" or "five heavenly animals," that give practitioners a powerful shamanic source of guidance, inspiration, and protection.

Once you become comfortable summoning these celestial guardians, you can use them to assist you whenever you need help in any area of your life: for example, if you are going through a troubling time, or if you find yourself frightened and needing support, or if you need a little extra inspiration. But really any time is a good time to access the power that these guardians represent. And the more you work with them, the more powerful they will become in your life.

To obtain the best results for the Dragon Gate dream yoga, we advise beginning with the practice of the five celestial guardians. This practice is also excellent for promoting positive energy and health for the organs associated with each guardian and it can be used as part of your five element practices outlined in the previous chapter.

FIVE CELESTIAL GUARDIANS EXERCISE

1. Find a comfortable place to stand. This can be inside or outside, but you should make sure that there are no major distractions such as noise, weather, etc.

2. Face north. If you do not know which direction north is, or if facing north is not practical for you based on your location, face the direction that is most appealing to you.

3. Close your eyes and take 3 deep breaths.

4. Visualize a green light emanating from your liver. (The liver is located in the right upper quadrant of your abdominal cavity, just below the diaphragm and to the right of your stomach.) Now visualize the green light moving from your liver, up through your torso, and out through your eyes where the light transforms into a green dragon that sits on your left side (outside of you).

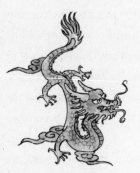

Green Dragon

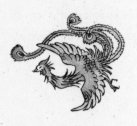

Red Phoenix

5. Visualize a red light emanating from your heart, moving up through your torso and out through your mouth where it transforms into a red phoenix floating above your head. (The phoenix is a sacred firebird from Chinese—and many other cultures'—mythology with fiery plumage. You can visualize the bird in any way that appeals to you.)

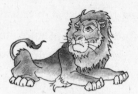

Yellow Lion

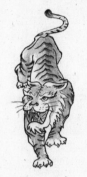

White Tiger

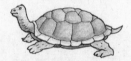

Blue Turtle

6. Visualize a yellow light emanating from your stomach, moving out through your navel, and transforming into a yellow lion in front of you.

7. Visualize a white light emanating from your lungs, moving up through your torso, and out through your nostrils where it transforms into a white tiger on your right side.

8. Visualize a dark blue light emanating from your kidneys. (You have two kidneys, which are located behind the abdomen, in the lower back area, one on each side of your spine.) Now visualize the blue light moving from your kidneys, up through your torso, and out through your ears where the light transforms into a blue turtle that stands behind you.

9. Once you have visualized all five celestial guardians, then say the following: "Great universal energy, honor the five celestial guardians and give me protection and wisdom."

10. Stand for a moment or two surrounded by your celestial guardians.

11. Now reverse the entire process. So visualize each celestial guardian (in reverse order: turtle, tiger, lion, phoenix, and dragon) turning back into light and the light returning to the organ from which it emanated, using the same path.

As you gain proficiency in manifesting the celestial guardians, you may summon them at any time for guidance, assistance, and protection. They can become a source of power and strength for you.

Note: If you have any difficulty at all in creating any of the visualizations in this exercise, simply imagine that you are doing it to the best of your ability.

DRAGON GATE DREAM PRACTICE

What follows is the core Dragon Gate dream yoga, which is comprised of several sections. They are meant to be done as a unit.

☯ Seven Stars

1. Make sure you are completely ready to go to sleep.
2. Stand in front of your bed and take 3 deep breaths.

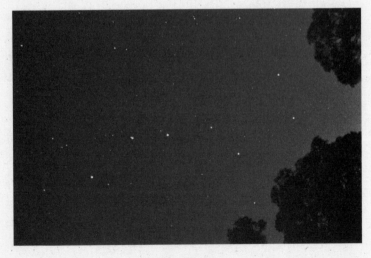

Big Dipper

3. Visualize the Big Dipper in the sky above your bed.

4. Bring the Big Dipper down to your bed so that you see the white points of light actually on your bed. Place the Big Dipper so that when you lie down on the seven stars your head is in the square. (When you eventually lie on your side your body should be in the same shape as the Big Dipper.)

☯ *Third Eye*

1. Once you have finished the seven stars practice, continue standing in front of your bed.

2. You will now do a series of clockwise and counterclockwise eye circles in 3 directions. To help visualize the circles use the visual metaphor of a clock. 1) The first direction is vertical circles to the side. For this you need to imagine your eyes circling vertically, that is, perpendicular to the ground and in line with your body (like the face of a clock that stands upright and faces to your front). 2) The second direction is horizontal. For this you need to imagine your eyes circling horizontally, that is, parallel to the ground (like the face of a clock that lies on its back facing up). 3) The third is vertical circles forward. For this you need to imagine your eyes circling vertically, that is, perpendicular to the ground and perpendicular to your body (like the face of a clock standing up and facing to your side).

3. Now look out through your third eye at the sky. (Visualize the sky above your bedroom.) Your third eye, according to Dragon Gate theory, is located between your eyes at the top of your nose.

4. At this point you may see a color or a light. If you do, think of yourself and the light as one.

5. Now bring your concentration to your navel and look out your third eye from the navel.

☯ Red Sun

1. Once you have finished the third eye practice, continue standing in front of your bed.

2. Now visualize yourself on a cloud, sleeping. A red sun rises in front of you.

3. Swallow the red sun, but keep it in your throat area and visualize it emanating a red light from your throat.

4. Now state the invocation to the red sun: "Great universal energy, help me to sleep like an angel and travel the heavens and the earth peacefully and harmoniously."

☯ Lie Down

1. Once you have finished the red sun practice, it is now time to get into bed.

2. Lie down on your side in the shape of the Big Dipper, which you had previously brought down to your bed. (You may

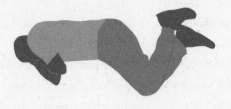

Dream

do this practice, lying on either side.) Place your bottom hand around the ear that is on the bed. Place your top hand on your bottom shoulder. The foot that is on top rests behind the bottom foot with the heel of the bottom foot resting on the top foot.

3. When you inhale contract slightly and when you exhale relax slightly.

☯ Conclusion: Dream Recall

1. Do this as soon as you wake up.

2. Stand up (or sit) and face east—the direction of the rising sun. (If you don't know which direction is east, face in the direction that feels best to you.)

3. Give yourself a "dry bath." Rub your palms together briskly 36 times, and then rub them over your face and body (as though washing yourself).

4. Ask yourself: what did I dream last night?

5. Make 3 deep sighs.

6. Take 7 deep breaths, filling your lungs completely and then exhaling quickly.

7. Place your consciousness in the third eye and visualize a white spark.

8. Cover your navel with both hands (men left hand on bottom, women right hand on bottom).

9. Continue recalling your dreams for as long as it feels productive. Then quickly write your dreams in your dream journal.

☯ Other Self

- Once you have become proficient in doing the dream practice outlined above, you can begin adding an advanced Taoist practice of the other self. To do this, while doing your dream practice, watch yourself doing the dream practice as though you are another person in the room.

Note: This exercise takes quite a bit of imagination. For instance, how do you look out of your third eye? Or how do you circle your eyes vertically? However, you will find that with a bit of practice your imagination will begin to easily conjure up these unusual ideas that are part of Dragon Gate dream practice. In addition, while it may take a bit of time when you start, once you become familiar with the practice you will be able to quickly run through it all in just a couple of minutes.

Dream Yoga Tips

Below are several suggestions for improving and enhancing your dream yoga practice.

AFFIRMATIONS
Here are several affirmations you can say to yourself as you are falling asleep.

- I remember my dreams.
- I awake in my dreams.
- I realize I am dreaming while I am dreaming.

- I am dreaming.
- I can control my dreams.

Feel free to try your own affirmations based on your experiences.

HERBS

Without recommending or endorsing any particular supplements, it is worth noting that many people find herbs helpful for dreaming. Herbs that have been used for millennia by people all over the world to enhance their dreams and dream recall include *Calea zacatechichi* (also known as the dream herb), *Silene capensis* (also known as African dream root), vervain, and licorice root.

WAKE YOURSELF

This suggestion is really only for those people who have the time and a flexible schedule that is suitable for this kind of practice, but interrupting your sleep cycle is a great way to stimulate lucid dreams and to aid your dream recall. The easiest way is to set an alarm clock to go off about an hour before you normally wake up. Then immediately go back to sleep. Another option is to use a clock to wake yourself up multiple times during the night and immediately go back to sleep. You will need to experiment with this method in order to find what works best for you and your system.

Here's to having bold adventures in your dream reality!

Seventh Gate: Dragon Gate Sexual Yoga

Using Dragon Gate Sexual Yoga for Energy Development and Spiritual Advancement

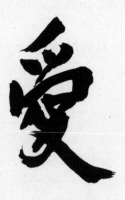

Love

One achieves longevity by loving the essence, cultivating the spiritual, and partaking of many kinds of medicines. If you don't know the ways of intercourse, taking herbs is of no benefit. The joining of man and woman is like the creation of heaven and earth.

—*The Canon of the Immaculate Girl,*
Ancient Taoist sexual manual

Please take a moment now to enjoy a brief moment of meditative contemplation before you proceed with this chapter. It will help you to maximize your enjoyment of the chapter.

Make yourself comfortable, close your eyes, and spend a few moments visualizing your partner in a perfect, radiant, energy-filled state of health and well-being. If you do not have a partner, then visualize yourself in this manner.

Now you are ready to begin.

Sexual Yoga

After they have concentrated and purified their thoughts, then a man and a woman may practice together the art that leads to longevity. This method allows a man and a woman together to activate their chi . . . And if this discipline is continued over a very long period, then it will become a natural habit and a method for living long and attaining immortality.

—DENG MING-DAO, *Seven Bamboo Tablets of the Cloudy Satchel*

For those fortunate enough to have a partner eager to pursue the magical path of Taoism, alchemical development can also be enhanced through the practice of Taoist sexual yoga. While there are ascetic schools of Taoism that eschew the use of sex as a vehicle for spiritual development, the use of sex as a method for cultivating chi and practicing internal alchemy are an integral part of Taoism. In fact, one of the legendary seven Taoist masters lived for a time in a brothel.

Taoist sexual techniques are an integral part of the inner alchemy and are referred to as "fang shu" or "fang zhong," which roughly translates to "inside the bedchamber" or "the art of the bedchamber." These practices involve "he chi," or "joining energy" or "joining essences." The theory is that by performing sexual yoga as part of a complete system of energy development, one can enhance health and even attain immortality.

Chinese alchemical principles are based on the idea that the universe and people are linked—that the microcosm of humankind is reflected in the macrocosm of the universe. Because of this, the concepts of yin and yang are as applicable to people as they are to the world around us. The overarching goal of Taoist sexual yoga is the union of yin and yang.

In the twenty-seventh century B.C., Huang Ti, the man credited with founding Chinese medicine, wrote in *The Yellow Emperor's Classic of Internal Medicine*: "I urge you to bring into harmony for me nature, heaven and Tao. There must be an end and a beginning. Heaven must be in accord with the lights of the sky, the celestial bodies, and their course and periods. The earth below must reflect the four seasons, the five elements, that which is precious and that which is lowly and without value—one as well as the other. Is it not that in winter man responds to yin? And is it not that in summer he responds to yang?"

According to Taoist philosophy, the passive and active principles of yin and yang are complementary parts of a greater whole. Health and longevity stem from a balanced interaction of yin and yang. The person who can maintain the balance by flowing with the cyclical currents of perpetual change is assured a healthy and long life.

Huang Ti wrote: "I have heard that in ancient times there were the so-called spiritual men, they mastered the universe and controlled yin and yang. They breathed the essence of life. They were independent in preserving their spirit. Their muscles and flesh remained unchanged. Therefore they could enjoy a long life, just as there is no end for heaven and earth. All this was the result of their life in accordance with the Tao, the right way."

From the Taoist perspective, sex between a man and a woman is an earthly manifestation of the universal principles of yin and yang. Consequently, long treatises and manuals have been written on how best to use sex to achieve the Taoist goals of health, longevity, and spiritual development. Among the Taoist "bedroom arts" classics that have been discovered are *Secrets of the Jade Bedroom*, *Chang San-Feng's Healing Techniques*, *The Sacred Manuscripts of Mt. Kung-Tung*, and *The Sacred Seal in the Heart*.

The content of these books has, for the most part, been kept secret for thousands of years. There is a long tradition in China of keeping advanced practices hidden and only passing them on to highly trusted disciples who have proven their loyalty over many years. In addition, the instructions in these manuals are written using metaphorical language to describe actual sex practices. For instance, the phallus may be referred to as the jade stem, the yang peak, or the ambassador, while the vagina may be referred to as the jade gate, the deep valley, or the celestial palace. The use of metaphors to pass on knowledge is another method of keeping information out of the hands of people who have not been properly initiated.

Nowadays this information is more readily available. And due to Western culture's strong interest in sex, information about sexual yoga and tantric sex has become so abundant that it is now difficult to know which information is accurate or appropriate.

Fortunately, the Dragon Gate system views sex as a normal part of life and includes many exercises and practices designed to simultaneously optimize the pleasure and metaphysical development of both lovemakers.

Please note that it is extremely important that both partners in a sexual relationship undertake the practice of sexual yoga together. When practiced correctly by two enlightened individuals, these exercises can lead to tremendous energy development for both people as well as a deeper spiritual relationship. However, when one of the partners is practicing sexual yoga techniques and the other partner is not, it can lead to serious imbalances in which the energy of the unaware partner can be drained. As with all techniques taught in this book, practicing with an open heart and positive intentions is a key element to achieving success.

The Vital Energy

Those seeking immortality must perfect the absolute essentials. These consist of treasuring the ching, circulating the chi, and consuming the great medicine.

—Ko Hung, fourth century Taoist alchemist

It's at this point that we come to an element of the Taoist alchemy that is often somewhat disturbing for men to contemplate. And that is that yin and yang are opposite forces of nature and they are not equal in all instances. In this case, successful use of sexual yoga requires that men control their ejaculations while women may have as many orgasms as they wish.

The reason for this is that, as outlined above, chi is the essential element in the Taoist alchemy and chi is developed from your ching (jing), or reproductive/sexual energy. So, when a man ejaculates, he ejects the essential ingredient in chi development. This idea is acknowledged by our modern culture in a number of ways. For instance, it is considered a truism in boxing that a fighter cannot have sex before a bout.

A man must devote a lot of energy to build up semen stores after an ejaculation. When the frequency of ejaculation exceeds the body's ability to replenish semen, men experience chronic fatigue, lower immune resistance, and feelings of irritation. Typically, in this instance, men also lose sexual interest in their partners.

The famous Taoist author Wu Shou-yang (ca. 1563–ca. 1632) wrote in *The True Principle Upheld by a Heavenly Immortal*:

> The great pass which divides life and death is the chi. The difference between a sage and an ordinary man is the ability to control the chi. Only by controlling the chi is one able to redirect the course of the sperm and convert it into the vital chi and to condense the spirit and diversify it into the vital spirit.

You may have heard of the medieval legend of the vampire-like female demon, known as a succubus, that comes to men (especially monks) in their dreams to seduce them. The succubus would use sex to drain energy from the men, often to the point of exhaustion or death, in order to sustain itself. The concept of the succubus was often used as an explanation for the phenomena of wet dreams and sleep paralysis.

Taoism also has its stories of succubus-like "fox" spirits that seek out followers of the Tao and drain them of all their vital energy. The necessity of preserving one's semen is a recurring theme in Taoist literature and philosophy.

On the other hand, when a woman orgasms, most of her sexual secretions are retained and reabsorbed within her own body. From the Taoist perspective this is a key reason why women, on average, live five to ten years longer than men.

The requirement for men to control ejaculations, however, is not the same as abstaining from sex. In fact, engaging in healthy sexual relations can increase the development of the chi, while abstaining from sex can cause physical and mental problems resulting from living out of harmony with nature and blocking the flow of chi.

The Classic of the Pure Lady is one of the essential manuscripts in the canon of Taoist sexology. It describes many methods that heighten, intensify, and prolong lovemaking. This book warns against celibacy: "Refraining from sexual intercourse is against nature. When yin and yang are not in contact, they cannot complement and harmonize each other . . . If a man can learn to control and regulate his ejaculations during sex, he may derive great benefits from this practice. The retention of semen is highly beneficial to man's health."

As with all aspects of Taoism, knowledge is the difference between success and failure. In the fourth century, the Taoist alchemist Ko Hung wrote: "If a man knows Tao, then the more he makes love, the better becomes his health. If he is ignorant of Tao, just one woman is sufficient to hasten his journey to the grave."

As part of the practice of sexual yoga men are encouraged to reduce the number of times their sexual encounters end in an ejaculation. There is no specific recommendation on the number of times a man should ejaculate. It is based largely on the health, vitality, lifestyle, environment, and the personal makeup of the individual. Typically, when a man notices how he feels after sex, he can determine how much is too much. The Taoists believe that optimum functioning occurs when actions flow in harmony with nature.

And while it may seem difficult to engage in sex without ejaculation, as you get better at it, you can achieve tremendous levels of satisfaction and pleasure combined with the ability to provide incredible fulfillment for your partner. This practice also has the added benefit of leaving a man feeling energized after sex, instead of spent. This does not mean that a man should never ejaculate, just that it should be controlled. In addition, whenever a man does ejaculate, ideally the loss should be compensated by absorbing the "essence" of the woman's secretions. Methods of doing this are described below.

For men who are wondering how there can be pleasure in sex without ejaculation, you may be comforted to know that the ancient Taoist masters asked the same question. In *Secrets of the Jade Bedroom*, Peng Tze, the sex adviser to the Yellow Emperor, wrote:

Question: It is generally assumed that a man gains great pleasure from ejaculation. But when he learns the Tao of yin and yang, he will ejaculate less and less. Will this not diminish his pleasure as well?

Answer: Not at all! After ejaculating, a man feels tired, his ears buzz, his eyes get heavy, and he longs for sleep. He is thirsty and his limbs feel weak and stiff. By ejaculating, he enjoys a brief moment of pleasure but suffers long hours of weariness as a result. This is no true pleasure! However, if a man regulates his ejaculations and retains his semen, his body will grow strong, his mind will clear, and his vision and hearing will improve. While a man must occasionally deny himself the fleeting sensation of ejaculation, his love for women will gently increase. He will feel as if he could never get enough of her. Is that not the true and lasting pleasure of sex?

According to this theory, the man who maintains high levels of ching and chi by practicing ejaculation control will experience greater love and affection for his partner and will also be able to make love to that woman as often as he likes, ensuring her complete satisfaction.

For the majority of men, completely abstaining from ejaculation can also be harmful because it is unnatural. It can lead to an obsessive desire for sex, which can cause both mental and physical blocks to energy development and can be self-defeating if the man ends up ejaculating during wet dreams instead. So every man has to figure out what works best for his own body.

The Taoist masters have provided different yardsticks for practitioners to use in gauging the number of acceptable ejaculations. Ultimately there is no one-size-fits-all approach since all alchemical practice is based on each individual's own particular makeup. For those of you who would like some guidance, the Yellow Emperor's adviser suggested the following: "Some men are strong, some are weak, some men are old and others are in their prime. Each should live according to his own vitality and not try to force the joys of sex." The advisor goes on to list the following suggestions for the frequency of sexual intercourse that ends in ejaculation:

Under age 20: unlimited
20–30 years old: 3–6 times per week
30–40 years old: 2–5 times per week
40–50 years old: 1–3 times per week
50–60 years old: 3–6 times per month

60–70 years old: 1–2 times per month

70+ years old: 0–1 times per month

But if you read a different text you will get different advice. Sun Simiao (also known as Sun Ssu-mo or the "Herbal King") was a famous doctor of the Tang dynasty (A.D. 618–907) who lived to the age of 101. A child prodigy, he became a well-known medical practitioner by the time he was twenty and was famous for his works on nutrition, health, and alchemy. When it came to ejaculation, Dr. Sun's basic recommendation was twice a month, or twenty-four times per year. His own personal regimen, however, was only one emission per one hundred sexual encounters.

A general guideline is that an ejaculation should leave a man feeling invigorated, not tired and uninterested in further sex. If an emission leaves a man feeling spent, he should increase the time between ejaculations.

Since women retain most of their own secretions when they orgasm, it doesn't result in the loss of their vital energy. Yet despite this key difference, the principles of Tao apply equally to men and women. In both, it is the "essence" of the reproductive fluids that is the key ingredient of the alchemy, which is why the successful retention, reabsorption, and channeling of these fluids is an essential element of sexual yoga.

A quick note on masturbation: From the Taoist perspective once a man has reached his twenties, he no longer has the seemingly inexhaustible supply of ching that he had in his teens and he should cease all masturbation and save his ching for his sexual relations. This proscription does not apply to women.

Exercises for Semen Retention and Groin Control

URINATION CONTROL

Taoists are known for taking normal elements of everyday life and turning them into opportunities for exercise, energy development, and spiritual growth. Consequently, they have devised a method of using the process of urination to aid in the training for sexual yoga.

These may be practiced by both men and women.

Holding the breath: During urination, hold your breath. If at first you cannot hold your breath during the entire process, hold it as long as you can and extend the period over time until you can hold your breath for a full urination. This will help to retain your chi.

Holding your talk: During urination, do not speak. This will help to retain your chi.

Holding the flow: During urination, break up the flow of the urine stream.

- Start with stopping the flow 3 times.
- Once you have mastered that, you can work on stopping the flow 9 times during a single urination.

This exercise greatly increases the strength of the muscles required to control ejaculation.

GROIN CONTRACTION

A key element in learning how to control ejaculation is gaining control over the muscles in the groin region. The following exercises do just that.

These may be practiced by both men and women.

There are three key points in the groin region. These are, from back to front, 1) the anus, 2) the perineum (the point directly at the bottom of the torso between the anus and the penis or vagina), and 3) the base of the penis or the vagina (the base of the urogenital canal).

This exercise may be practiced standing, sitting, or lying down.

1. Contract the anus 3 times.
2. Contract the perineum 3 times.
3. Contract the base of the penis or the vagina 3 times.
4. Contract all three points simultaneously 3 times.

If at first you have trouble isolating the muscles in these regions, don't worry. This is common. Start off by visualizing the point and the contraction and do the best you can. After some practice you will gain much better control. Once you are comfortable doing 3 contractions, work your way up to 9.

GROIN CONTRACTION DURING SEX

Men may use variations of the groin contraction (described above) during intercourse to stop ejaculation or to help minimize the loss of energy when they choose to ejaculate. Women may use these variations to increase both their own and their partner's pleasure during sex and to retain more of their own sexual secretions.

During sex: Practice the groin contraction during sex. For men, this can be used to stem the flow of sperm and prevent ejaculation. You can choose to do any of the three points separately or together. As you do this exercise, visualize (and feel) the energy rising from your groin, up your spine, and to your brain.

After ejaculation: Approach ejaculation slowly by moderating your pace and breathing deeply. Just as you are reaching climax, use the groin contraction method to contract and hold each of the three points simultaneously. Continue to practice the groin contraction exercise for a minute or two after ejaculation.

This exercise helps to reduce the amount of chi lost by men during ejaculation and it helps women as well by helping them to prevent the loss of chi.

HOLDING THE BREATH

You can use breath-holding as another method of preventing ejaculation. When you feel yourself approaching climax, simply hold your breath for a count of 9. You may also combine this with the groin contraction exercise.

MIND LINKING

One of the best methods of preventing premature orgasms is by linking the mind to the sex act. This enables you to stop the process that leads to orgasm at will. It takes a bit of practice to master this technique, but if you practice it, you will succeed.

While engaged in sex, focus your mind on your groin.

Now withdraw the mental focus from the groin and bring it up to your brain.

Repeat this process multiple times.

CONTRACTING

While engaging in sex, the man can mentally withdraw and cause his penis to contract. Once the level of penile excitement has reduced, the man can resume his previous mental state.

When men choose to use any of these exercises to prevent ejaculation, it is important that their partner be aware of and agree to what they are doing so that they are not made to feel left out or abandoned in the process. As with all sexual yoga techniques, the involvement of and open communication between both parties is essential to achieving optimal results.

Taoist Sexual Relations

The King sent the woman to ask P'eng the Methuselah about the ways of prolonging life and benefiting old age. Said P'eng, "Heaven and earth have attained the methods of intercourse and therefore they lack the limitation of finality. Man loses the method of intercourse and therefore suffers the mortification of early death. If you can avoid mortification and injury and attain the arts of sex, you will have found the way of nondeath."

—*The Canon of the Immaculate Girl*

In order for a man to sexually satisfy his partner and to foster energy development, he must learn to extend the duration of intercourse. Once men learn to control their ejaculations they and their partners can gain tremendous benefits from sex.

For men, sexual yoga consists of suppressing emissions, absorbing the woman's fluids, and retaining semen to strengthen the mind and body in order to attain longevity and enhanced mental capabilities. For women, sexual yoga consists of achieving climax as often as possible, retaining their own sexual secretions, absorbing the man's secretions when he chooses to ejaculate, and using these sexual fluids to strengthen the mind and body in order to attain longevity and enhanced mental capabilities.

As a general guideline, for women, frequent intercourse with orgasm is the key to the successful practice of sexual yoga. For men, frequent intercourse with infrequent ejaculation is the key. The practice of semen retention enables a man to reabsorb his own essence, and it also lets him prolong sex so his partner can reach orgasm and release her own sexual fluids, which he can absorb as well.

The key to sexual yoga is the interplay of yin (female) and yang (masculine) energies. As noted in *Classic of the White Madam*:

> For a man to nurture his male powers, he must nourish his yang essence by absorbing yin essence. When men and women indulge freely in sex, exchanging their bodily fluids and breathing each other's breath, it is like fire and water meeting in such perfect proportions that neither one defeats the other. Man and woman should ebb and flow in intercourse like the waves and currents of the sea, first one way then another, but always in harmony with the great tide. In this manner, they may continue all night long, following the basic harmony of yin and yang constantly nourishing and preserving their precious vital essence, curing all ailments, and promoting long life.

Viewing the sexual yoga on a purely biochemical level, the sexual secretions of both men and women contain many hormones, enzymes, and proteins. When female secretions are released during sex they are absorbed by the skin of the man's penis. Likewise, the woman's vagina also absorbs these same emissions as well as the man's semen after he ejaculates inside her. The hormones and other substances in the sexual fluids are then circulated throughout the man's and woman's body and affect the various systems that manage the health, vitality, and energy of the individual.

In the ideal sexual encounter, the man waits for his partner to climax and then spends some time absorbing her energy and sexual fluids with her. Then, if he feels that he has enough energy to share, the man ejaculates himself so both partners absorb each other's sexual essence and energy.

It's also worth noting that while a man's energy secretions come primarily from his sperm, according to Taoist literature, a woman releases essence that is useful for sexual yoga from her tongue and nipples in addition to the vagina, and men can benefit from all three. In *Secrets of the Jade Bedroom*, Peng Tze points out: "During intercourse, if a man takes in a lot of the woman's saliva, it will purify his stomach like medicinal broth." The same is true for the nipples and vagina, but it is important to remember that this is only true once the woman has been sufficiently aroused.

Foreplay

> Not only should the male element be nourished, but the female element should likewise be.
>
> —*Secret Instructions Concerning the Jade Bedroom*

Taoist sex manuals typically advise a period of foreplay at the beginning of the sex act. This is used to raise the energy levels of both men and women and to ensure sufficient female lubrication and male erection prior to sex.

EYE GAZING EXERCISE FOR COUPLES

The following exercise can be used by couples as a form of foreplay or as an exercise to do at any time that will further deepen and develop your relationship. Repeated practice of the eye gazing exercise continually yields new insights into your partner and yourself. The benefits of this exercise to enhance a spiritual relationship cannot be overestimated.

- Both partners should find a comfortable place to sit where the lighting is subdued and you can directly face each another. This can be inside or outside, but you should make sure that you can sit comfortably for a period of time and that there are no major distractions such as noise, weather, etc., that could disturb your meditation. It's a good idea to turn off the phone and anything else that may bother your practice.
- The lighting needs to be low enough that you can comfortably keep your eyes open for a long period of time.
- Ideally, you should sit facing each other on the edge of a hard chair with your backs not touching the back of the chair. Your feet should be on the floor and your knees should be bent at an approximately 90-degree angle. However, if you would prefer, you can choose to sit in any other configuration as long as you can sit comfortably for a period of time and you can easily face each other. Other possibilities include sitting cross-legged on the floor, or sitting on a sofa or at a table.
- Make sure you are wearing something loose and comfortable.

If you are wearing a belt, undo it. If your skirt or pants have a tight waistline, open them.

- During this exercise breathe through your nose and keep your tongue on the roof of your mouth, just behind the upper teeth, with your teeth lightly touching.

1. Close your eyes, relax, and take 3 deep breaths, filling and emptying your lungs completely each time.
2. Open your eyes and gaze into the eyes of your partner.
3. Continue gazing into your partner's eyes for as long as it is comfortable. Blink as often as you need to, but the longer you can go without blinking the better.
4. Practice eye gazing for a minimum of 5 minutes, however, you can practice much longer if you wish. (You may set a timer to monitor the amount of time you spend, however, it is important that the timer alarm sound is soft and melodious, so that you are not disturbed by it when it goes off.)

EROTIC MASSAGE

An excellent way to maximize the pleasure of lovemaking is to begin with an erotic massage prior to intercourse. The erotic massage should start at the body's extremities and then should slowly progress to the genitals. The massage can be given by one partner to the other or by both partners to each other simultaneously. It is important to study your partner and learn from his or her responses which points are most stimulating and generate the most energy.

1. Start by massaging the hands and wrists.
2. Work your way up the arms and shoulders.

3. Move to the feet and ankles.

4. Then massage up the legs and thighs.

5. Now move to the back and shoulders.

6. Next massage the chest and abdomen.

7. Finally massage the genital areas.

Couple Sexual Yoga Exercises

SYNCHRONIZING THE BREATH

In this exercise the man and the woman synchronize their breathing, with both partners breathing in and out at the same time. Keep your tongue on the roof of your mouth, just behind your upper teeth. You may also synchronize the movement of the sexual act to coincide with the breathing. The couple should avoid breathing directly on each other to ensure the intake of plenty of fresh air. As you do this exercise, visualize (and feel) the energy rising from your groin, up your spine, and to your brain.

FAST AND SLOW METHODS OF INTERCOURSE

The man alternates fast and slow thrusts. The alternation helps the man to avoid premature ejaculation, which prolongs the sex act and raises the energy level.

In fast, out slow: As the man thrusts in, he should move quickly. As he withdraws the penis, he should move slowly. During the slow withdrawal, the man should focus on absorbing as much of the woman's sexual fluids as possible.

In slow, out fast: As the man thrusts in, he should move slowly. As he withdraws the penis, he should move quickly. During the slow insertion, the man should focus on absorbing as much of the woman's sexual fluids as possible.

LONG AND SHORT METHODS OF INTERCOURSE

Short and long: The man alternates short (incomplete) and long (deep) thrusts. The alternation helps the man to avoid premature ejaculation, which prolongs the sex act and raises the energy level.

3 short–1 long: The man does 3 short thrusts followed by 1 long thrust.

9 short–1 long: The man does 9 short thrusts followed by 1 long thrust.

GROIN CONTRACTION FOR COUPLES

Both men and women can practice the groin contraction exercises outlined earlier in this chapter. These exercises help both men and women to prolong the sex act, increase the energy level, and prevent the loss of energy. They are especially important for a woman to practice after she and/or the man have climaxed in order to retain as many of the sexual secretions as possible.

PRIMING THE PUMP

Both men and women can use the groin contraction exercises to swell and contract the penis and vagina during sex. In this way both the man and the woman can increase their pleasure and the absorption of their partner's sexual secretions.

RIDING THE WAVE

This exercise requires that both the man and the woman reach the verge of climax together. Just as they are both on the verge of climax they should stop, with the man keeping his penis inside the woman. The couple should maintain as much skin contact as possible by embracing. Each partner should focus on raising the energy up their spines from their groins to their heads. After a few moments, when the height of excitement has subsided, the couple should begin again, and may repeat this process as many times as they enjoy. This practice should be engaged in only once the man has attained a good degree of ejaculation control.

DRAWING OUT

The man should mentally draw the energy (chi) from the tip of the penis back to the base of the spine and up the spine to the head. The woman should mentally draw the energy (chi) from the vagina back to the base of the spine and up the spine to the head. As the chi continues to gather in the groin region, both partners should continue this process.

UNITING AT ORGASM

According to the theories of sexual yoga, there is a burst of energy when a man or woman reaches orgasm. Partners may absorb each other's energy as follows:

Breathe fresh air: Avoid breathing in the breath of your partner at the moment he or she orgasms. You can keep your head nuzzled under your partner's ear or turn your head to the side.

Embrace your partner: It is important to maintain maximum skin contact during orgasm as energy radiates from the entire body.

Press the pubic regions closely together: The biggest burst of sexual energy during orgasm occurs in the pubic region and the greatest benefits are achieved by keeping the pubic regions close together.

Couples may practice any or all of these exercises during any given sexual encounter. It is advisable to start off slowly, attempting to practice one or two of these exercises and work your way up.

Eighth Gate: Wealth and Manifestation

SIMPLE AND INTUITIVE DRAGON GATE MANIFESTATION PRACTICES BASED ON YIN AND YANG AND THE YI JING

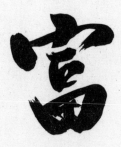

Prosperity

The ingenuity of that which causes material form is patent to the eye, and its operations are superficial. Therefore it arises anon, and anon it vanishes. Only one who knows that life is really illusion, and that death is really evolution, can begin to learn magic.

—LIEH TZU, FIFTH CENTURY B.C.

Please take a moment now before you begin this chapter to practice this brief and simple exercise. It will help you to maximize your enjoyment of the chapter.

Find a place where you are completely comfortable.

Spend a few minutes feeling gratitude. You may feel gratitude for anything you wish that is a part of your life.

Now you are ready to begin.

Manifestation

When I let go of what I am, I become what I might be.

—LAO TZU

One of the central tenets of Taoism is that reality is a projection of consciousness, and many Dragon Gate exercises are designed to guide you to a state where you can experience this for yourself. Because reality is a thought construct, by focusing the mind, perfecting concentration, and practicing visualization, you can become conscious of the ways you have manifested the reality you are currently experiencing and also gain the ability to change that reality in accordance with your own thoughts, desires, and will.

Consequently, a basic goal of Dragon Gate Taoism is assisting seekers on the path to manifest the means to achieve their goals. At a basic level, what you manifest is the result of choices you have made. Change your choices and you will change what you manifest. Choose to eat well and exercise and your health will improve. Choose to do unhealthy things and your health will suffer.

However, manifestation also works on a much more complex level. After all, who wouldn't choose to manifest health, wealth, spiritual fulfillment, deep and rich relationships and a life filled with rewards of every kind? The simple fact is that everyone manifests a wide variety of experiences. From a Taoist perspective this is done in order to experience many ways of being, and while we may not manifest everything that we believe we want according to our conscious preferences, it is important to honor and respect all of our manifestations as a product of our own unique creativity.

In an effort to assist its practitioners, Dragon Gate has developed numerous tools to aid the process of manifestation. To begin understanding the Dragon Gate concepts of reality projection and manifestation, it is useful to understand their ideas on how the universe we experience comes into being.

Yin and Yang

One Yin and one Yang, this is the Tao.

—BOOK OF CHANGES

Everyone is very familiar with the Taoist yin/yang symbol.

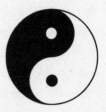

This represents the two fundamental forces of nature, described as yin and yang.

However, before there was yin and yang, according to Taoist philosophy, in the beginning there was only void, known as wu-chi, which is typically represented as an empty circle.

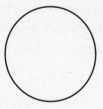

This void represents a state of unity and nondifferentiation. In other words, in the wu-chi state there is only void and nothing else. But this void contains the potential for the creation of everything because without void there is no room for anything else to emerge. This concept is captured in a famous Zen story called "A Cup of Tea":

> A pompous university professor visited a Zen master to question him about the nature of reality. The master served the professor tea, and poured it into the professor's cup until it overflowed and spilled on the floor.
>
> "You have overfilled the cup," the professor exclaimed. "There is no more room."
>
> The master replied, "Like this overflowing cup, you are too full of your own ideas. There is nothing I can teach you, until you empty your cup."

In other words, in order to fill anything up, or to create, there must first be a space for that creation. This is why the first step in manifestation is to create the space for that which you desire to bring into existence.

From the void emerged yin and yang, the opposite forces of nature that brought into existence the dualistic reality we experience on a day-to-day basis. Reality is dualistic because everything we perceive is defined in terms of its opposite. For instance, there would be no hot without cold, no light without dark, no large without small, no love without hate and so on.

> Being and non-being create each other.
> Difficult and easy support each other.
> Long and short define each other.
> High and low depend on each other.
> Before and after follow each other.
>
> —LAO TZU

So yin and yang represent the two primary forces of the universe and in Taoist theory everything is assigned either a yin or yang nature, or a combination of the two. For instance, the earth is yin while heaven is yang, night is yin while day is yang, water is yin while rocks are yang, etc.

Typically yang energy is viewed as light, fast, active, solid, hot and hard, while yin is viewed as dark, slow, passive, diffuse, cold, and soft. It is important to remember that there is no judgment assigned to these forces of nature. Neither is better than the other. They are complementary forces that are mutually dependent. Moreover, they always work as a pair and strive to attain a balance in natural harmony, which is the Taoist ideal. As depicted in the yin/yang symbol both yin and yang arise and then transform into the other in a never-ending fluid and circular cycle. The dot of the opposite color that sits within each of the black-and-white swirls represents the idea that each of the two forces contains the seed of the other force within it.

The importance of the concepts of void and the yin and yang that arise from the void cannot be overstated. They are at the core of most Chinese philosophy and are an integral part of every aspect of Chinese society including philosophy, medicine, art, cooking, and martial arts.

CREATING THE VOID EXERCISE

> The world is formed from the void, like utensils from a block of wood.
> The Master knows the utensils, yet keeps to the block.
> Thus he can use all things.
>
> —LAO TZU

The first step in manifestation is creating the space in which to manifest that which you desire. This exercise is designed to assist you in that process.

1. Find a comfortable place to sit or lie down. This can be indoors or outside, but make sure that there are no major distractions such as noise, weather, etc.
2. Close your eyes and take 3 nice, deep breaths.
3. In your mind, create a completely empty space. This space can be as large as you want. Use whatever metaphor works for you as a symbol of empty space, such as outer space.
4. In your mind, position yourself at the outer edge of that empty space.

5. Now invite into that empty space whatever it is that you would like to manifest in your life.

6. Observe what emerges in the space. Do not attempt to judge or edit what manifests. Simply think about what it is that you would like to manifest and watch what occurs.

7. Observe and notice the manifestation arising, stabilizing, and then dissolving. Make no effort to affect this process. Simply allow it to unfold. If you have judgments or thoughts about the process such as "I like this" or "I don't like that" simply observe those thoughts as well but make no effort to suppress or develop them further.

8. Spend 3 to 5 minutes doing this practice. If nothing emerges, don't worry about it. That is fine. If that occurs, simply observe the empty space. This will make you more comfortable with the concept of void and the process of creating the space required for manifestation.

Yi Jing

The Changes is a book from which one cannot hold aloof. Its Tao is forever changing, alteration, movement without fixed law, firm and yielding transform each other. They cannot be confined within a rule; it is only change that is at work here.

—BOOK OF CHANGES

In order to manifest that which you desire, it is essential to make the best decisions possible, since what we experience is the result of the choices we make. This is why Chinese philosophy has devoted a great deal of thought and energy to devising methods for divining the best path to take in any given situation. The culmination of this thinking can be found in the Yi Jing (I Ching), or "Book of Changes," which is one of the most important books in Chinese philosophy.

The Yi Jing, which takes its name from *yi*, which means "change," and *jing*, which means "classic" or "book," is both a philosophical treatise explaining how the universe functions and a divination manual that represents the evolution of the binary system embodied in the concepts of yin and yang. It's important to remember that all the exercises and theories in this book—including the divination practices in this chapter—are derived from the precepts outlined in the Yi Jing and so it is useful to understand what the Yi Jing is and a bit of its history.

On a philosophical level, the Book of Changes affirms the life-giving, creative nature of the Tao in which harmony between heaven, earth, and human can only occur through adaptability to a state of perpetual change. It is by successfully adjusting to the constant change that exists in life that one becomes a more successful conscious creator.

The Yi Jing outlines three fundamental principles:

• Follow the simple: This refers to idea that the appropriate course to follow in most situations in life is obvious. For instance, eat when you are hungry, sleep when you are tired, do unto others as you would have done to yourself, etc. Of course, people can superimpose complex interpretations on simple situations that turn the easy into the difficult. So in order to manifest we need to return to the basic simplicity of life. When confronted with any situation we should first consider the simplest solution. This idea was summed up by Confucius when he wrote: "The way out is through the door. Why is it that no one will use this method?"

- Everything changes: In life we can expect that everything changes. We get older each day and our bodies and minds are in a constant state of flux. The world around us also appears to constantly change. Ideas that were once held to be truth suddenly become obviously false, and fringe concepts become accepted facts. So when we want to manifest we need to take advantage of the way that everything is always changing. This enables us to know that when things are not going our way, we can expect our situation to change. Similarly, when things are going well we can prepare for the inevitable change to come in order to achieve the best result from it. This is why the Yi Jing states: "When the way comes to an end, then change. Having changed, you pass through."

- Everything stays the same: Just as we can see that everything changes, on another level, we see that everything stays the same. In other words, there are general patterns that repeat. There are always four seasons and 365 days in a year, 28 days in a lunar cycle, 24 hours in a day, and so on. These patterns repeat in ways that are completely predictable. So we need to be cognizant of that which is foreseeable in our lives and use it to our best advantage. This is why the Yi Jing states: "One should act in consonance with the way of heaven and earth, which is enduring and eternal. The superior man perseveres long in his course, adapts to the times, but remains firm in his direction and correct in his goals."

By the way, it is inherently Taoist to marry two completely diametrically opposed ideas—such as everything changes and everything stays the same. This mirrors the yin and yang forces of the universe.

To fashion a divination manual out of this philosophy, ancient Chinese thinkers codified a theory on the laws of the universe and the flow of time, space, and energy by combining yin and yang elements into three-part ideograms known as "guas." The resulting eight trigrams represent the eight possible ways of combining yin and yang in a three-line structure. In the trigrams (and hexagrams of the Yi Jing), yin is symbolized by a broken line and yang is symbolized by a solid line.

The trigram is a binary expression of the core Chinese philosophical view of the world as divided into heaven (the top line),

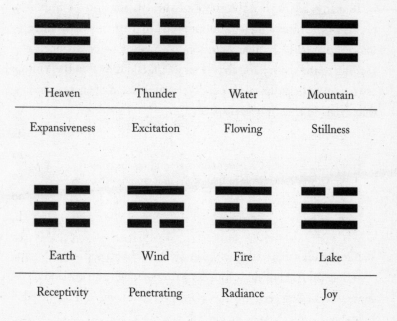

Heaven	Thunder	Water	Mountain
Expansiveness	Excitation	Flowing	Stillness

Earth	Wind	Fire	Lake
Receptivity	Penetrating	Radiance	Joy

The eight guas, their name, and their basic energy pattern.

human (the middle line), and earth (the bottom line). Then, by combining two guas, a new system of sixty-four six-line patterns were formed, creating the sixty-four hexagrams of the Yi Jing.

According to the legend, the Yi Jing was written by the mythical founder of Chinese civilization, Fu Hsi, five thousand years ago when he saw the eight trigrams on the back of a turtle that emerged from a river. Later, in the twelfth century B.C., King Wen, while in prison after being captured by an evil adversary, studied these original trigrams and developed the hexagram system by doubling them. It is believed that he gave each figure a name and description. Then his son added commentary to form the core of the Yi Jing text we know today. By the time of Confucius (ca. 500 B.C.) the Yi Jing had become an integral part of Chinese philosophy.

It seems likely that the roots of the Yi Jing can be found in prehistoric Chinese divination methods that were revised and enhanced over time by many authors. Whatever its provenance, according to the theory, the sixty-four changes outlined in the Yi Jing are meant to describe every possible combination of energy pattern that exists in this time and space.

> The ancient Chinese mind contemplates the cosmos in
> a way comparable to that of the modern physicist.
>
> —CARL JUNG

While the idea that reality as we know it can be parsed into a binary system comprised of sixty-four set patterns may seem outlandish to some, the Yi Jing certainly has a devoted following, not only in the East, but in the West as well.

The Yi Jing initially came to the West in the late seventeenth century when a Jesuit, Joachim Bouvet, who had been working in China, brought the book to Gottfried Wilhelm Leibniz, the renowned German mathematician who was one of the inventors of calculus as well as the binary system upon which all computer programming is based. Leibniz was fascinated that the ancient Chinese had created a binary system capable of expressing any possible value. To him, this showed how God could create the universe from unity and nothingness. He wrote: "As far as I understand, I think the substance of the ancient theology of the Chinese is intact and can be harnessed to the great truths of the Christian religion. Fu Hsi, the most ancient prince and philosopher of the Chinese, had understood the origin of things from unity and nothing, i.e., his mysterious figures reveal something of an analogy to Creation, containing the binary arithmetic (and yet hinting at greater things) that I rediscovered after so many thousands of years, where all numbers are written by only two notations, 0 and 1."

Carl Jung is another famous Western thinker who was fascinated by the Yi Jing and saw it as a metaphor for his own ideas on archetypes and synchronicity. Jung thought that "whoever invented the Yi Jing was convinced that the hexagram was the exponent of the moment in which it was cast." This coincided with his belief that "synchronicity takes the coincidence of events in space and time as meaning something more than mere chance, namely, a peculiar interdependence of objective events among themselves as well as with the subjective (psychic) states of the observer or observers."

More recently, a fascinating correlation between the Yi Jing and DNA, the fundamental building block of life, has been discovered. The Yi Jing describes sixty-four possible permutations to describe what manifests in our reality. The double-helixed structure of our

DNA is composed of four types of base pairs: thymine, adenine, cytosine, and guanine. Three of these base pairs make an amino acid and together are called a triplet. This, of course, correlates to the yin/yang trigrams. But even more intriguing is that there are sixty-four possible combinations of these base pairs. The synchronicity is striking.

Divination

The future can be seen right now. Because the future is made of the present. If you look deeply into the present, you know already what kind of future you'll have.

—THICH NHAT HANH

Whether or not the ancient Chinese figured out the fundamental structure of life from the markings on the back of a mythological tortoise is only as relevant to you as you make it. As Jung himself points out, "The Yi Jing does not offer itself with proofs and results; it does not vaunt itself, nor is it easy to approach. Like a part of nature, it waits until it is discovered. It offers neither facts nor power, but for lovers of self-knowledge, of wisdom—if there be such—it seems to be the right book. To one person its spirit appears as clear as day; to another, shadowy as twilight; to a third, dark as night. He who is not pleased by it does not have to use it, and he who is against it is not obliged to find it true. Let it go forth into the world for the benefit of those who can discern its meaning."

Since the Yi Jing provides metaphorical answers, it is not designed to be used with yes and no questions. Rather, the greatest benefit is meant to be found by asking for guidance and direction. This is true for all types of divination. Ultimately, the power of decision making is one of the greatest treasures we possess and it is not advisable to hand that power over to any other source whether it's a person or a five-thousand-year-old divinatory technology. The answers you receive are a reflection of your own consciousness and help you to choose a wise and fruitful path.

What follows are two very simple Dragon Gate divination exercises that you can practice at any time when you would like insight into the path you should follow. As with the Yi Jing, we advise not selecting yes and no questions. Seek guidance and direction from these exercises—not specific answers. Also, remember that the information will often come to you in a metaphorical way that will require you to be open to it in order to receive it and then interpret it correctly.

DRAGON GATE WATER DIVINATION EXERCISE

1. Before you go to sleep at night, fill a glass of water and put it by your bedside.
2. Focus your mind on a strongly held wish or question. It can be anything that is important to you.
3. Hold the glass of water in your hand and energize the water with your question or wish. Now drink half the glass of water. Then lie down and go to sleep.
4. In the morning, the first thing you should do when you wake up is drink the other half of the glass of water.
5. Pay attention to what happens to you during the course of the day as you should receive information that helps you to answer your question or choose which direction to follow in order to fulfill your wish.

DRAGON GATE DREAMING
DIVINATION PRACTICE

This is a very simple divination technique that you can use with the Dragon Gate Dream Yoga practice described in Chapter 6.

1. Purchase a piece of "special" yellow paper. It can be any kind of paper, but just make sure it is special to you—that is, a kind of paper you do not normally use or buy.
2. Write a strongly held wish or question on the yellow piece of paper. Fold the paper 5 times (to invoke the power of the five elements).
3. Place the paper under your pillow.
4. Do the Dragon Gate Dream Yoga practice (from Chapter 6).
5. Note any dreams you have within the seven days after doing this practice as the dreams should help you to answer your question or choose which direction to follow in order to fulfill your wish.

The Third Eye

Many teachers will tell you to believe; then they put out your eyes of reason and instruct you to follow only their logic. But I want you to keep your eyes of reason open; in addition, I will open in you another eye, the eye of wisdom.

—SRI YUKTESWAR

Another method for developing intuition and insight into choosing the optimal path to your goals is the development of the third eye. According to the theory, which is common to virtually all esoteric traditions, the third eye, also known as the inner eye or eye of wisdom, represents a portal to inner realms and higher consciousness. It is also strongly associated with clairvoyance, visions, out-of-body experiences and other metaphysical phenomena.

While the specific location of the third eye varies somewhat among different belief systems, it is generally placed between the eyebrows at the sixth, or brow, chakra. In Taoist alchemy it is the location of the upper dantian (tan-tien). And though it is a psycho-spiritual organ in humans, other species, such as reptiles and amphibians, actually have a physical third "parietal" eye that is able to sense light and is believed to assist in regulating circadian rhythms and navigation, among other things.

Many spiritual writers and philosophers associate the third eye with the pineal gland, a small endocrine gland about the size of a pea and shaped like a tiny pine cone (from which it derives its name) that is located in the center of the brain between the two hemispheres. While the functions of the pineal gland are not completely understood, it is known to produce melatonin, a hormone that affects our circadian rhythms. The gland is believed to play a role in our sleep cycles, sexual development, and metabolism. On a metaphysical level, the pineal gland is typically associated with the development of psychic abilities. René Descartes, the seventeenth-century mathematician and philosopher who coined the phrase "I think therefore I am," called the pineal gland the "seat of the soul," whose primary function was "to receive the psychic spirits"—in other words, it was a connecting link between the physical and spiritual worlds.

Practices involving the use of the third eye are common throughout Eastern mysticism, including Dragon Gate. As you may have noticed, it is part of the dream yoga practice outlined in Chapter 6.

Dragon Gate Third Eye Practice

Dragon Gate Taoism has developed techniques designed to stimulate the third eye and the intuitive abilities associated with it. This is a simple and powerful exercise you can do by itself or in conjunction with other exercises detailed in this book.

1. Find a comfortable place to sit or stand. This can be indoors or outside, but make sure that there are no major distractions such as noise, weather, etc.

2. Assume your posture, close your eyes, and take 3 nice, deep breaths.

3. Visualize three bright white points of light in front of you on the same line. At the microcosmic level these three points of light represent the left eye, the right eye, and the third eye. At the macrocosmic level they represent the sun, the moon, and the pole star.

4. Now move the three points of light toward you until they sit directly over your two physical eyes and the third eye located in between them.

5. Now allow the white lights on your two eyes to converge on the point of light in the center (over your third eye). Focus your attention on the white light at your third eye. Hold the light there for 2 to 3 minutes.

6. Now, with your eyes still closed, look through your third eye at the open sky above you. (If you have any trouble "looking" through your third eye, simply imagine what it would be like.) Do this for 2 to 3 minutes.

7. When you are ready to complete the practice, rub your palms together briskly 36 times, and place them lightly over your

eyes. (The palms should "cup" the eyes so that no light gets in and you can feel the heat from your palms, but the palms do not touch your eyelids.) Palm your eyes for a minute.

The best way to tell if your mental abilities are growing is if you notice an increase in the number of "coincidences." According to Dragon Gate theory, there are no coincidences, but when you perceive them to be happening, you are actually witnessing your own powers of conscious creatorhood being unveiled for you. So pay close attention to them.

From the Taoist perspective, "coincidences" are simply our becoming aware of our union with everything—our oneness with the Tao. This idea is very similar to the Jungian concept of synchronicity. Jung was very fond of telling a story passed on to him by Richard Wilhelm, the famous translator of the I Ching, that he felt perfectly explained this idea:

There was a catastrophic drought in Kiao-chau, where Wilhelm lived. The Catholics paraded, the Protestants prayed, and the Chinese burned joss-sticks and shot off guns to frighten away the demons of the drought. But still the rain did not come. Finally the Chinese said, "We will fetch the rain-maker."

And from another province an old man appeared. The only thing he asked for was a small, quiet house where he could meditate for three days. On the fourth day the clouds gathered and there was a great snow-storm at a time of the year when no snow was expected. Naturally curious, Wilhelm went to ask the man how he did it. He said: "Will you tell me how you made the snow?" And the Chinese man said, "I did not make the snow, I am not responsible."

"But what have you done these three days?"

"Oh, I can explain that. I come from another country where things are in order. Here they are out of order. They are not in Tao, and so I also am not in the natural order of things because I am in a disordered country. So I had to wait three days until I was back in Tao and then naturally the rain came."

Creating the Right Circumstances

If you do not change direction, you may end up where you are heading.

—LAO TZU

This chapter began with a discussion of how objects in physical reality manifest from the void and how to create a space in which to create that which you desire. Next we looked at methods for selecting the right path to choose using divination techniques and methods designed to promote your intuition. The next step in the process of conscious manifestation involves creating the optimal circumstances for your manifestation to appear. Taoism has created its own metaphysical science dedicated to just that process, which is called feng shui.

Feng shui (literally "wind and water") is the ancient Chinese art of placement—or how to arrange your environment to create optimal circumstances for your health, wealth, and happiness. A useful metaphor for thinking about how feng shui works is to think of a nail and a magnet. If you place a nail on a magnet, the previously nonmagnetized nail becomes magnetized by its proximity to the magnet. Similarly, your environment contains numerous factors that exert an energetic influence over you when you spend a great deal of time in that environment. So, by adjusting the environment in order to open blockages, alleviate stress points, and improve the flow of energy, you can create a more beneficial environment for yourself.

Dragon Gate offers some very simple techniques that can be used by anyone at any location to create a more harmonious space at any time. The best of this type of practice is the Five Guardians feng shui. This method uses the traditional feng shui "magic square," a 3 x 3 grid that looks like a tic-tac-toe grid. The Chinese name for this grid, Lo Shu, is derived from the myth surrounding its creation, which is that the original magic square appeared to the legendary patriarch of Chinese civilization, Fu Hsi, on the back of a turtle that emerged from the river Lo. The magic square is also part of the Yi Jing divinatory tradition, which uses the following configuration.

The Magic Square

4	9	2
3	5	7
8	1	6

There are numerous interesting numerological elements in the magic square that contribute to its reputation. A quick look reveals how the grid is arranged so that the five odd numbers form a cross through the center of the square while the four even numbers are at the corners. If you add up three numbers in any direction, the total is fifteen, which corresponds to the number of days in each of the twenty-four cycles of the Chinese solar year.

The sectors of the magic square also relate to the eight trigrams that form the basis of the sixty-four hexagrams used in the Yi Jing, the five elements, as well as actual physical directions. In this way the magic square can be mentally placed over whatever location you want to perform the Five Guardian feng shui practice on. Using the traditional magic square, north is placed at the bottom (at 1), but for the purposes of our brief divination exercise, we will use the bottom as the front of your location. In a house this would be the side facing the street. You can also apply this to your own office within a larger building. In that case the front door would be the 1 (bottom) location.

DRAGON GATE FIVE GUARDIANS FENG SHUI

To do the Dragon Gate Five Guardian feng shui, do the following:

1. Place yourself in the feng shui location. Lie down, sit, or stand in a place that is as close to the center of your location as you can comfortably arrange. Position yourself so that you are facing the street or front of your location.
2. Close your eyes and take 3 deep breaths.
3. Visualize the magic square over your location, aligning the bottom with the street or front of your location.
4. **Green Dragon:** Visualize a green light emanating from your liver and moving from your liver, up through your torso, and out through your eyes where the light transforms into a green dragon that sits in the left side quadrant of your location. Visualize a green light filling the location.
5. **Red Phoenix:** Visualize a red light emanating from your heart, moving up through your torso, and out through your mouth where it transforms into a red phoenix that floats in the air in the front quadrant of your location. Visualize a red light filling the location.

6. **Yellow Lion:** Visualize a yellow light emanating from your stomach, moving out through your navel, and transforming into a yellow lion in the central quadrant of your location. Visualize a yellow light filling the location.

7. **White Tiger:** Visualize a white light emanating from your lungs, moving up through your torso, and out through your nostrils where it transforms into a white tiger in the right quadrant of your location. Visualize a white light filling the location.

8. **Blue Turtle:** Visualize a dark blue light emanating from your kidneys and moving from your kidneys, up through your torso, and out through your ears where the light transforms into a blue turtle that stands in the rear quadrant of your location. Visualize a dark blue light filling the location.

9. When you are done, the mental configuration of your location should be like this:

	Blue Turtle	
White Tiger	Yellow Lion	Green Dragon
	Red Phoenix	

Front

10. Now say the following: "Great universal energy, honor the five celestial guardians and purify the energy at this location."

11. Now reverse the entire process. So visualize each celestial guardian (in reverse order: turtle, tiger, lion, phoenix, and dragon) turning back into light and the light returning to the organ from which it emanated, using the same path.

Knowing When to Act

Opportunities multiply as they are seized.

—SUN TZU

If you have created the space for manifestation to occur, chosen the best path, and optimized your circumstances, you must still know the optimal time to act. In other words, you have to have good timing as well. Taoism addresses this with the concept of wu wei.

Wu wei literally means "not doing." However, as with many ideas in Chinese philosophy, the words require a metaphorical translation in order to grasp the true meaning. A more useful translation of wu wei is "effortless doing," which means acting in accordance with the Tao, or in harmony with nature. So just as the sun revolves around the earth and rivers flow into the sea, in ideal circumstances your actions will flow naturally with the circumstances to create the outcome you desire.

In practical terms this means that while you may be able to achieve a goal under any circumstances, if your actions are in harmony with the natural cycles it will be far easier to attain. Often this translates to waiting for the right moment—choosing wisely— rather than acting impulsively. Ideally, if you have created the proper circumstances for yourself, you may be able to achieve your result without taking any obvious action.

One way to use wu wei in your process of manifestation is to play out your ideas of manifestation on a mental level. The following exercises will help you to do that.

DRAGON GATE VISUALIZATION FOR MANIFESTATION EXERCISE

Visualization is one of the most powerful techniques available for manifesting what it is that you want to bring into your life. Since Taoism holds that reality is a thought construct, everything occurs on the mental level before appearing in physical reality. You can use visualization to work on manifesting any positive experience you desire in your life.

1. Find a comfortable place to sit or lie down. This can be inside or outside, but you should make sure that there are no major distractions such as noise, weather, etc.

2. Contemplate what it is that you would like to manifest. Choose something that you feel strongly about.

3. Close your eyes and take 3 deep breaths.

4. Now visualize yourself in the state of having manifested that which you desire. Visualize as many details as possible. Where are you? What are you wearing? What are you doing? What is the weather? What does the air smell like? Are there objects involved, and if so, what do they look and feel like? Attempt to activate all five of your senses in this visualiza-

tion. Spend several minutes with this visualization or more if you feel like it.

5. Now spend several minutes creating a strong feeling of trust within yourself that this manifestation is real—as real as the ground that supports you.

6. Now shift your focus to the feelings of pleasure you have from your manifestation. Feel both the physical and the emotional pleasure you feel from attaining your goal. Focus on the pleasure for several minutes.

7. Now shift your focus to a feeling of gratitude for the manifestation. Spend several minutes feeling gratitude for what it is that you are manifesting.

DRAGON GATE MANIFESTATION
BILOCATION EXERCISE

The bilocation exercise allows you to develop skills in manifestation by enabling your consciousness to easily shift between perspectives and realities.

1. Find a comfortable place to sit or lie down. This can be inside or outside, but you should make sure that there are no major distractions such as noise, weather, etc.

2. Think about where you are now and what it is that you perceive yourself lacking. Then think about what it is that you would like to manifest (choose something that you feel strongly about).

3. Close your eyes and take 3 nice, deep breaths.

4. Now visualize yourself in the state of having manifested that

which you desire. Visualize as many details as possible and activate as many senses as you can in this visualization in order to make it as real as possible. Spend 1 to 2 minutes in this state.

5. Now shift your consciousness to where you perceive yourself to be lacking and visualize that as clearly as possible (in as much detail and activating as many of your senses as possible). Spend 1 to 2 minutes in this state.

6. Now shift back and forth from each of these two poles of experience. Spend approximately 1 minute in each pole of your bilocation and continue shifting as long as you desire, but visit each pole a minimum of three times.

DRAGON GATE SEXUAL YOGA MANIFESTATION PRACTICE

There is a very simple wish fulfillment technique that you can use in conjunction with the sexual yoga techniques described in Chapter 7. The idea behind this exercise is to use the energy you can generate with sexual yoga and alchemize that energy into the world to manifest what it is you desire. Make sure you have the agreement and cooperation of your sexual partner before engaging in this exercise.

1. Choose an event for which you want a successful outcome. This could be an important business meeting, the launch day for a new product, a job interview, and so on.

2. For the week prior to the event date, abstain from having sex.

3. On the seventh night—the night before the event—engage

in sex and achieve climax. Prior to having sex, focus on the event that is coming the next day and visualize the positive outcome that you desire.

Final Thoughts on Manifestation

The superior person contains the means in his own person. He bides his time and then acts.

—BOOK OF CHANGES

Manifestation is a tricky skill. Even those people who are the best at it find themselves regularly manifesting things in their lives that do not appear to be in line with their conscious preferences. This is because reality functions on many levels, and we choose to bring an assortment of elements into our lives in order to fulfill a variety of complex experiences that are all part of being a human being.

If you are having difficulty manifesting that which you desire, or you are unhappy with what you find in your life, try not to be upset. It is what you have chosen to experience for some reason that you may not be aware of. As a guide to your manifestation abilities, you can look at what is in your life—because whatever you are experiencing is something you are manifesting. So if you are having any problems, avoid asking yourself "Why am I creating this?" and instead ask yourself "How am I creating this?" This question is a key that opens the powerful door of conscious manifestation.

Another important point to remember is that according to Dragon Gate philosophy, the physical realm is guided by the rules of karma. The development of your ability to create the reality you wish also carries responsibilities, because each and every action has an equal and opposite reaction. Consequently, the ability to manifest also requires an understanding of karma. So the various tools outlined in this chapter may only be used to benefit yourself and not to hurt anyone or anything else. Attempting to use these techniques to hurt others is likely to result in harm to yourself. It is also advisable that if you encounter success you share some of it with those around you who are less fortunate. This keeps the cycle of energy flowing.

Ninth Gate:
Advanced Alchemy

EASY WAYS TO INTEGRATE THE ESSENCE OF DRAGON GATE INTO YOUR DAILY LIFE

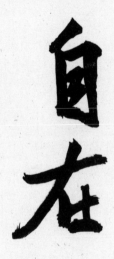

Freedom

To conduct one's life according to the Tao is to conduct one's life without regrets; To realize that potential within oneself which is of benefit to all.

—LAO TZU

Please take a moment now before you begin this chapter to practice this brief and simple exercise. It will help you to maximize your enjoyment of the chapter.

Find a place where you are completely comfortable.

Spend a few minutes thinking about a coincidence you have experienced recently. If you have any difficulty coming up with one, try again another time.

Now you are ready to begin.

Now You Are Ready to Begin

If one desires to cultivate the path of immortals, one must first cultivate the path of men. As long as the path of men has not yet been cultivated, the path of immortals will be far.

—WANG CHONG-YANG, A FOUNDER OF COMPLETE
REALITY TAOISM, TWELFTH CENTURY A.D.

You have now reached the final chapter of this particular journey into the world of Dragon Gate Taoism. This chapter is called "Advanced Alchemy," but in actuality the entire book is filled with advanced alchemical practices from the Dragon Gate tradition that have been put into a format that makes them safe and accessible to anyone. So what makes this chapter "advanced"? In typical Taoist fashion the answer lies in returning to the beginning.

A key to getting the most out of Dragon Gate Taoism is to find ways of incorporating the philosophy and practices into your day-to-day life. After all, what is the benefit of learning a potentially life-changing system of meditation, philosophy, exercise, and magic, if you cannot find the time to practice it? It is a fundamental truth of all physical and metaphysical practice that regular, steady practice—even in very small amounts—is superior to long periods of practice done infrequently. So I would advise you to incorporate those exercises and techniques that appeal to you into a regular program that is easy for you to make a part of your daily life.

This book is filled with easy exercises that you can practice in just a few minutes a day. If you have more time, do more, but do your best to do something every day—even if it is only for a couple of minutes. It can be helpful to incorporate practices into a ritual. So, just as you brush your teeth when you wake up and before bed, you can find exercises that are easy for you to do at particular times of the day.

When you integrate the essence of Dragon Gate into your daily life you will find that it provides you with greater clarity, well-being, relaxation, stamina, and enjoyment of every aspect of your life. It is also a great way to break up a stressful day—take a few minutes to meditate or do a breathing exercise. You will also find that the more you practice, the easier it is to do and the greater the results.

You can start with just one or two exercises from the book, then add in more and replace the ones you have done to get a feeling for what all the practices offer you. The ones that particularly appeal to you can become part of a regular regime. Others you may use for only a brief time.

It is by making these exercises a part of your daily life that you truly begin to create a magical Taoist reality.

Simplicity

I have just three things to teach: simplicity, patience, and compassion. These three are your greatest treasures.

Simple in actions and in thoughts, you return to the source of being.

Patient with both friends and enemies, you accord with the way things are.

Compassionate toward yourself, you reconcile all beings in the world.

—LAO TZU

While we may sometimes believe that something that is complex is superior to something that is simple, when it comes to metaphysical practices, the opposite is often what is true. That's why Dragon Gate has developed many very easy and simple practices that you can incorporate into your daily life.

DRAGON GATE NUMBERS

Dragon Gate has a unique number-reciting method to promote health and wellness. It is based on the eight trigrams with the idea that it is a mirror of the eight cranial bones of the human brain (see Chapter 8). Reciting each number creates a specific brain wave that affects your mental functioning, which in turn affects the physical functions.

To use these, simply say the number to yourself silently (this is very important—*do not speak the number aloud*). You can recite these numbers (silently, to yourself) in any language (but you should say them in your primary language).

ISSUE	NUMBER TO RECITE MENTALLY	APPLICATION
Sleep	6030	When lying down to sleep to make you fall asleep
Losing Weight	7788	Before a meal for a minute to curb appetite
Wake Up / Alertness	4050	Any time you haven't gotten enough sleep or need to be alert, such as driving at night
Sex	65030	During sex to promote stamina
Focus	10	Any time you need focus
Meditation	1060	Any time you are meditating this calms the mind
Stamina	6503080	Before and during exercise
Constipation	60	Just before and during a trip to the bathroom

Another valuable method for incorporating Dragon Gate practice into a busy schedule is to use simple techniques that are done in conjunction with your normal day-to-day activities.

DRAGON GATE WALKING PRACTICE

Walking is something almost everyone does every day. Whether it's for exercise or just to go from our parking spot to your office, we often spend time walking. Usually we spend that time engrossed in thoughts or chatting on our cell phones. But we can also use that time to practice Dragon Gate.

1. Before you begin your walk, take one deep breath and as you exhale mentally say the word *relax* and feel your mind and body relaxing.

2. Now mentally prepare yourself for your Dragon Gate walk by reminding yourself that you are going to walk with the intention of practicing Dragon Gate. This should take no more than 1 to 2 seconds. Now tell yourself, "As I walk with each step I take, I will get closer to achieving my goals."

3. Now begin your walk. As you walk, while you may cross different terrain and various obstacles, do your best to keep your gait and pace steady. As you walk, focus on your breathing and do your best to breathe slowly, deeply, and regularly.

4. To focus your mind you can count your breaths or say the meditation number described above.

5. You can use this any time you are walking, no matter what the duration or distance.

Important note: Only do this practice in a situation that is completely safe—places where you do not have to worry about traffic or dangerous situations, etc.

DRAGON GATE FOOD PREPARATION PRACTICE

Preparing food and eating is another thing you do every day. Even if you do not cook, you can take the time that you prepare to eat (washing your hands, choosing your food, spreading a napkin, picking up your silverware, and so on) to do this exercise.

1. Before you begin preparing your food or getting ready to eat, take one deep breath and as you exhale mentally say the word *relax* and feel your mind and body relaxing.

2. Now mentally prepare yourself for your Dragon Gate food practice by setting your intention to practice Dragon Gate. This should take no more than 1 to 2 seconds. Now tell yourself, "The food I am preparing (or the food I am about eat) will nourish me and provide me with the energy and nutrients I need to achieve my goals."

3. Now begin preparing your food or preparing to eat. As you do this, focus on your breathing and do your best to breathe slowly, deeply, and regularly.

4. To focus your mind you can count your breaths or mentally say the meditation number described above.

5. Do this practice as long as you desire. If there are others around, remember that they will not know what you are doing, so you may want to keep the duration of the exercise short.

DRAGON GATE WASHING PRACTICE

Washing in all its myriad forms (bathing, showering, washing hands, brushing teeth, etc.) is another activity we do every day that can be used to promote your Dragon Gate practice.

1. Before you begin washing take one deep breath and as you exhale mentally say the word *relax* and feel your mind and body relaxing.

2. Now mentally prepare yourself for your Dragon Gate washing practice by setting your intention to practice Dragon

Gate. This should take no more than 1 to 2 seconds. Now tell yourself, "As I wash myself, I am cleaning away anything that may be holding me back. When I emerge cleansed I will be closer to achieving my goals."

3. Now begin washing. As you do this, focus on your breathing and do your best to breathe slowly, deeply, and regularly.

4. To focus your mind you can count your breaths or say the meditation number described above.

5. Do this practice as long as you desire.

You may use these simple daily practices as a basis for incorporating Dragon Gate into your other daily activities.

The Factors of Life

> It is only when we have the courage to face things exactly as they are, without any self-deception or illusion, that a light will develop out of events, by which the path to success may be recognized.
>
> —BOOK OF CHANGES

If you are reading this book, chances are you are working on improving the quality of your life—typically in numerous areas including spiritual, health, employment, relationships, and financial. This book provides practices designed to assist you in all those areas. But as part of the process of improving and enhancing your life, it is also good to do a mental accounting of the various aspects of your life in order to determine where you are doing well and where you need to place more energy in order to achieve the results you desire.

According to Dragon Gate philosophy there are numerous factors that guide your success in life. The factors are:

- **Fate**: This is what you are born with, including your physique, family, location, time in history, base health, and so on. While your fate is not something you have conscious control over, the way you feel about it is in your control. And this is critical. If you view your fate from the perspective of victimhood ("why was I handed this lot in life?") that sense of victimhood will permeate your entire life. So it is very important to seek out the positive. This does not mean you should sweep things under a mental rug. It means that you change your orientation toward any aspects of your "fate" that you view negatively from one of victimhood to one of being involved in the creation of your fate as part of your experience on this earth. Good and bad things happen to all of us, but you are not a slave to how you choose to react to those events. You always have free will in terms of how you respond mentally to any situation and Dragon Gate encourages you to enjoy and revel in your free will and make the most of it.

- **Life Pass**: Your life pass is what you have done with your life. In other words, it is the choices you have made. Where have you gone? What have you done? Who have you chosen to associate with? How have you invested your time? It is important to look at your life pass and determine if you are happy with the choices you have made and, if not, to take steps to remedy the situation as soon as possible by making new and different choices.

- **Feng Shui**: As described earlier in this book, feng shui is the art of placement—or optimizing your environment to enhance your opportunities. Look at where you live and where you spend your time. Do you feel that the location is conducive to achieving your goals or is it hindering them? What can you do to improve where you live? What can you do to improve where you work? Do you need to move to a better location?

- **Good Deeds:** Taoism embraces the concept of karma. You reap what you sow. Or to put it in the language of physics, every action has an equal and opposite reaction. Consequently, you can improve your life by doing good deeds, which includes everything from helping others to cleaning the environment. Interestingly, numerous studies have shown that altruism is as beneficial to the person doing the good deeds as to those receiving the direct benefits. If you feel there is something missing in your life, try volunteering one day a week (or whatever you have time for). You may be surprised at who benefits the most.

- **Learning:** One of the most powerful things you can do in your life is learn. Learning opens up doors to amazing new thoughts and realities for you. There are numerous benefits to study, which include enhanced mental function, improved job qualifications, and experiencing greater enjoyment of life. It is important that you keep learning throughout your life. And while metaphysical studies are very important, you should also try something new. Feed your sense of wonder and curiosity. It is an essential aspect in your growth.

- **Discipline:** In order to achieve your goals, you need the discipline to follow your path. Discipline applies to every aspect of our lives including health, work, and spiritual practice. If you find discipline a challenge, the important thing to remember is to start small and stay focused. As noted above, it is better to do a small amount of practice (or whatever it is that you wish to do) every day than to do a large amount all at once. Make your practice a habit and find ingenious ways to stick with it.

- **Health:** Good health is a very important part of following the Tao. That is why Taoism places such emphasis on good health and includes so many techniques for promoting energy and longevity. Naturally, some people are born with better health than others. However, no matter what your natural gifts, you can optimize your physical health through exercise, diet, chi gung, and meditation.

- **Rest:** While work and discipline are important in determining whether you achieve your goals, so is knowing when to take a break. If you find that you are stressed out, take a vacation. If you find that you are no longer progressing on the path you are following, take some time off. To paraphrase a famous general, when you take some time to regroup and restore you're not retreating, you're advancing in a different direction.

- **Attitude:** Whatever happens to you in your life, your attitude about the occurrence will be the most important factor in how it affects you. To reiterate the famous quote from the Yi Jing: "The auspicious and the ominous both arise from the same circumstances." A key way to ensure that you maintain an optimal attitude is to maintain your health, energy, and mental focus.

- **Decisions:** The decisions you make and the actions you take (see the next factor) are ultimately the greatest source of personal power that you have in your life. So it is important to fully engage in the decision-making process and enjoy the power it represents. In addition, once you make a decision, you must act on it.

- **Actions:** The actions you take (based on the decisions you make) will be the single most important factor in determining where you end up in life. Action is what causes everything to occur. However, it is important to know when and how to take action. To do this, you need to develop your intuition, learn to trust yourself, and practice. Taking action, like everything else in life, becomes easier and the results improve with practice.

The essence of incorporating Dragon Gate practice in your daily life involves successfully managing these factors and following the natural rhythm, or to use traditional Taoist language, living in accord with the Tao. And if you find the idea of exploring every aspect of your life a bit daunting, try thinking of it as an adventure and break the process down into the smallest pieces you require to feel comfortable. Remember, these concepts and practices are meant to empower you, not to cause stress or doubt. If you do have those feelings, relax and do some breathing exercises. Dragon Gate is about adding fun and pleasure to your life. Enjoy it.

Dragon Gate Healing Techniques

> The person who possesses the source of enthusiasm will achieve great things. Doubt not. You will gather friends around you as a hair clasp gathers the hair.
>
> —BOOK OF CHANGES

Another form of advanced alchemy is helping others, and one of the best ways to do that is through mental and physical healing. Transforming pain and suffering into comfort and joy is truly an amazing alchemical process. That is why Dragon Gate has an entire medical system based on developing a free flow of chi, acupuncture, and herbal medicine. While most of the techniques are quite advanced and require years of study before you can use them to assist others, there are a couple of very simple methods you can use right away.

Note: Please be aware that these techniques are only to be used for very mild issues that do not require professional medical attention.

Dragon Gate Vital Palm Energy Technique

This is a simple exercise you can use with a friend to help them any time they feel depressed or have low energy, or notice that they have a mild illness coming on (such as a cold).

1. Have your friend sit in a chair while you stand beside him or her. You should both remain silent and breathe deeply during this practice.
2. You and your friend should both take 3 deep breaths.
3. Rub your hands together vigorously 36 times (your palms should feel hot).
4. Place your left palm over your navel.
5. Place your right hand 2 to 4 inches above the head of your friend.
6. Focus your mind on the positive thoughts, such as love, good health, and happiness that you wish to send to your friend.
7. Do this for 1 to 2 minutes.

☯ *Alternate Method for Long Distance*

- If the friend you wish to help is not in the same location, then take a few moments to get a clear picture of your friend in your mind. Then hold your right hand up and visualize sending the energy to them.

Note: You must only send positive thoughts with this exercise, because negative thoughts will negatively affect you.

DRAGON GATE PALM HEALING TECHNIQUE

This is a simple exercise you can use with a friend to help them alleviate any minor aches and pains they may have.

1. You and your friend should both take 3 deep breaths.
2. Have your friend lie down on his or her stomach on a bed, a couch, a mat, or a carpeted floor as long as it's comfortable and there is room for you to sit beside him or her.
3. You should both remain silent and breathe deeply during this practice.
4. Starting at the bottom of your friend's spine, hold your palm in the air approximately 1 inch above the spine.
5. Close your eyes.
6. Slowly move your hand up your friend's spine (no more than 1 inch every 5 seconds of so). Mentally project energy from your palm toward your friend's back. At any point along the spine where you feel a blockage in the energy flow, pause and hold your palm over this spot until you feel the energy flowing again. The energy may be perceived as heat or a sensation of tingling, or a magnetic force.

7. Move your hand along the spine until you reach the neck. Then move back down to the base of the spine.

8. If you have any difficulty sensing any blockages, don't worry about it. Move your hand back and forth (slowly) along the spine up to 3 times. If you still don't feel anything, try again another time.

Advanced Taoist Alchemy Energy Development Exercises

> There must be some primal force, but it is impossible to locate. I believe it exists, but cannot see it. I see its results, I can even feel it, but it has no form.
>
> —ZHUANG ZI

In previous chapters, you learned a wide variety of Dragon Gate energy development exercises. These are designed to create a free flow of chi within the body, which is the first step in the internal alchemy process.

The following advanced alchemical exercises are designed specifically for the further refinement of energy.

THE MICROCOSMIC ORBIT EXERCISE

One of the more powerful energy development exercises in all of Taoism is known as the microcosmic orbit. This involves circulating the energy around the body in a prescribed pattern.

The following is a brief synopsis of *The Secrets of Cultivation of Essential Nature and Eternal Life*, written by the Taoist master Chao pi Ch'en (born 1860): "Taoist alchemy focuses on the cultivation of the sexual and reproductive force. The force is kindled by regulated breathing and directed into the microcosmic orbit. The course of the orbit starts at the base of the spine, the first gate, rises up the spine to the second gate, between the kidneys, and then to the back of the head, called the third gate, before reaching the brain. The energy is then brought down the face, chest, and abdomen to return to the base of the spine, hence completing a full circuit."

Find a comfortable place to sit. This can be inside or outside, but you should make sure that you can sit comfortably for a period of time and that there are no major distractions such as noise, weather, etc., that could disturb your meditation. It's a good idea to turn off the phone and anything else that may disturb your practice.

As with all sitting exercises we recommend that you sit on the edge of a hard chair with your back not touching the back of the chair. Your feet should be on the floor and your knees should be bent at an approximately 90-degree angle. Make sure you are wearing something loose and comfortable. If you are wearing a belt, undo it. If your pants have a tight waistline, open them.

During this exercise breathe through your nose and keep your tongue on the roof of your mouth with your teeth lightly touching.

1. Close your eyes, relax, and take 3 very deep breaths, filling and emptying your lungs completely each time.
2. Breathe in: As you breathe in feel the energy rising from the point at the base of your spine, rising up your back and along the spine until it reaches the top of your head. Breathe slowly and evenly so you complete an entire in breath as the energy rises.
3. Breathe out: Now begin to breathe out and feel the energy

slowly dropping down the central line in the front of your body, across your face, chest, and abdomen, until it comes to rest once again on the base of the spine. Your exhalation should complete just as the energy reaches the bottom of your spine.

4. Repeat this process 9 times. If you are short on time you can do it 3 times and if you are particularly enjoying it you may practice the orbit 36 times.

THE GOLDEN STOVE EXERCISE

In Taoism the alchemical process is often compared to a metallurgical process in which fine metals are refined in a burning stove of energy. This particular exercise is extremely powerful and is an excellent way to alleviate pain and help the body's natural healing processes.

Find a comfortable place to sit. This can be inside or outside, but you should make sure that you can sit comfortably for a period of time and that there are no major distractions such as noise, weather, etc., that could disturb your meditation. It's a good idea to turn off the phone and anything else that may disturb your practice.

As with all sitting exercises we recommend that you sit on the edge of a hard chair with your back not touching the back of the chair. Your feet should be on the floor and your knees should be bent at an approximately 90-degree angle. Make sure you are wearing something loose and comfortable. If you are wearing a belt, undo it. If your pants have a tight waistline, open them.

During this exercise you breathe through your nose and keep your tongue on the roof of your mouth with your teeth lightly touching.

1. Close your eyes, relax, and take 3 deep breaths, filling and emptying your lungs completely each time.

2. Rub your lower back with your palms in small circles 36 times.

3. Now visualize a fire burning at the base of your spine and filling your entire body with heat and energy.

4. Now feel the energy move to the energy center at your navel (known as the lower dantian). Take 3 deep breaths, making sure to breathe slowly, deeply, and evenly, and with each deep breath, feel the energy at your navel growing and being heated by the fire at the base of your spine.

5. Now feel the energy move to the energy center at the solar plexus (known as the middle dantian). Take 3 deep breaths, making sure to breathe slowly, deeply, and evenly, and with each breath, feel the energy at your solar plexus growing and being heated by the fire at the base of your spine.

6. Now feel the energy move to the energy center in your head, between your eyes (known as the upper dantian). Take 3 deep breaths, making sure to breathe slowly, deeply, and evenly, and with each deep breath, feel the energy at your head growing and being heated by the fire at the base of your spine.

7. Now take 3 more deep breaths and feel the energy you have accumulated spread throughout your entire body.

Conclusion

The ancients understood that life is only a temporary sojourn in this world and death is a temporary leave. In our short time here we should listen to our own voices and follow our own hearts. Why not be free and live your own life?

—Lieh Tzu

We hope that you have enjoyed this brief sojourn into the world of Dragon Gate. We have done our best to provide you with the most valuable information that you can learn on your own without a teacher on hand to assist you. Many of the practices explained in this book have never been in print before and truly are secrets of the Dragon Gate system.

The book is not meant to be all-encompassing or complete. It is an overview of what Dragon Gate has to offer and we encourage you to take from it that which most appeals to you. We deeply hope that the book in some small or large way adds to your enjoyment of life and your understanding of yourself and the reality you find yourself in.

And in conclusion we would like to wish you bold flowing in the adventure that is your life.

It is never too late to become what you might have been.

—George Eliot

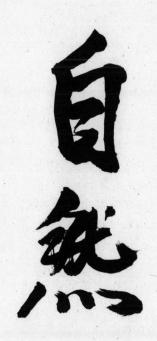

Nature

ACKNOWLEDGMENTS

We thank our families (Marion, Martin, and Colby in particular), our teachers, our friends, and our students. Without their help, guidance, and support we would have never discovered the secrets of Dragon Gate. We also thank our publisher, Tarcher/Penguin, Michael Solana, Joel Fotinos, and the entire team who brought this book into the world. In addition, we thank our indefatigable literary manager, Peter Miller.

ABOUT THE AUTHORS

Dr. Steven Liu grew up in Taiwan and began studying Taoism as a boy. In his twenties, he met White Crane, the thirteenth Master of the Dragon Gate school of Taoism in Taiwan. After many years of study and passing a series of rigorous trials, Dr. Liu became the fourteenth-generation master of the system.

Dr. Liu is a graduate of Hu-Bei College of Chinese Traditional Medicine and is a licensed acupuncturist, currently seeing patients and developing new healing herbs and technologies at his Golden Life Acupuncture Center in Los Angeles, California.

For more information, visit www.goldenliving.us.

Jonathan Blank is an award-winning writer, filmmaker, and creative technologist. He has spent more than twenty-five years studying high-level martial arts, meditation, Eastern philosophy, and esoteric metaphysical practices with many remarkable teachers in the United States, Asia, and Europe.

Blank took the first steps on his Taoist journey as a teenager and has continued along that path to this day. In 1996, he met Dr. Liu and has been learning and practicing Dragon Gate Taoism ever since.

Blank has a B.A. and an M.F.A. from Columbia University in New York.

For more information, visit www.jonathanblank.com.